Immunology at a Glance

KT-232-006

Immunology at a Glance

J. H. L. PLAYFAIR

Emeritus Professor of Immunology
Royal Free and University College Medical School
London

B. M. CHAIN

Professor of Immunology
Royal Free and University College Medical School
London

SEVENTH EDITION

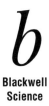

**Blackwell
Science**

© 1979, 1982, 1984, 1987, 1992, 1996, 2001 by
Blackwell Science Ltd
Editorial Offices:
9600 Garsington Road, Oxford OX4 2DQ
25 John Street, London WC1N 2BS
23 Ainslie Place, Edinburgh EH3 6AJ
350 Main Street, Malden
  MA 02148-5018, USA
54 University Street, Carlton
  Victoria 3053, Australia
10, rue Casimir Delavigne
  75006 Paris, France

Other Editorial Offices:
Blackwell Wissenschafts-Verlag GmbH
Kurfürstendamm 57
10707 Berlin, Germany

Blackwell Science KK
MG Kodenmacho Building
7–10 Kodenmacho Nihombashi
Chuo-ku, Tokyo 104, Japan

Iowa State University Press
A Blackwell Science Company
2121 S. State Avenue
Ames, Iowa 50014-8300, USA

The right of the Authors to be
identified as the Authors of this Work
has been asserted in accordance
with the Copyright, Designs and
Patents Act 1988.

All rights reserved. No part of
this publication may be reproduced,
stored in a retrieval system, or
transmitted, in any form or by any
means, electronic, mechanical,
photocopying, recording or otherwise,
except as permitted by the UK
Copyright, Designs and Patents Act
1988, without the prior permission
of the copyright owner.

First published 1979
Reprinted 1980
Italian edition 1981
Second edition 1982
Reprinted 1983 (twice)
Spanish edition 1983
Third edition 1984
Fourth edition 1987
Japanese edition 1987
Reprinted 1988, 1990, 1991
Fifth edition 1992
Four Dragons edition 1992
Japanese edition 1993
Chinese edition 1994
German edition 1995
Sixth edition 1996
International edition 1996
Seventh edition 2001
Reprinted 2001, 2003

Set by Best-set Typesetter Ltd., Hong Kong
Printed and bound in Great Britain
by MPG Books Ltd., Bodmin, Cornwall

The Blackwell Science logo is a
trade mark of Blackwell Science Ltd,
registered at the United Kingdom
Trade Marks Registry

DISTRIBUTORS

Marston Book Services Ltd
PO Box 269
Abingdon, Oxon OX14 4YN
(*Orders*: Tel: 01235 465500
        Fax: 01235 465555)

USA
  Blackwell Science, Inc.
  Commerce Place
  350 Main Street
  Malden, MA 02148-5018
  (*Orders*: Tel: 800 759 6102
          781 388 8250
    Fax: 781 388 8255)

Canada
  Login Brothers Book Company
  324 Saulteaux Crescent
  Winnipeg, Manitoba R3J 3T2
  (*Orders*: Tel: 204 837 2987)

Australia
  Blackwell Science Pty Ltd
  54 University Street
  Carlton, Victoria 3053
  (*Orders*: Tel: 3 9347 0300
        Fax: 3 9347 5001)

A catalogue record for this title
is available from the British Library

ISBN 0-6320-5406-9

Library of Congress
Cataloging-in-publication Data

Playfair, J.H.L.
    Immunology at a glance /
    J.H.L. Playfair, B.M. Chain. —7th ed.
      p. ; cm.
    Includes bibliographical references and index.
    ISBN 0-632-05406-9
    1. Immunology.   2. Immunology—Charts,
    diagrams, etc.   I. Chain, B.M.   II. Title.
    [DNLM: 1. Immunity—Terminology—English.
    QW 540 P722i 2000]
    QR181.P53 2000
    616.07'9–dc21   00-044446

For further information on
Blackwell Science, visit our website:
www.blackwell-science.com

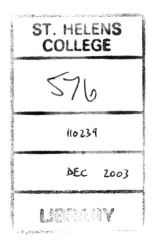

ST. HELENS
COLLEGE

576

110239

DEC 2003

LIBRARY

Contents

Preface 6
Acknowledgements 6
Note on the seventh edition 6
How to use this book 7
Further reading 7

Immunity
1 The scope of immunology 8
2 Natural and adaptive immune mechanisms 10
3 Evolution of immune mechanisms 12
4 Cells involved in immunity: the haemopoietic system 14

Natural immunity
5 Complement 16
6 Acute inflammation 18
7 Phagocytic cells: the reticulo-endothelial system 20
8 Phagocytosis 22

Adaptive immunity
(i) The cellular basis
9 Lymphocytes 24
10 Primary lymphoid organs and lymphopoiesis 26
11 Secondary lymphoid organs and lymphocyte traffic 28

(ii) The molecular basis
12 Evolution of recognition molecules — the immunoglobulin superfamily 30
13 The major histocompatibility complex 32
14 The T cell receptor 34
15 Antibody diversification and synthesis 36
16 Antibody structure and function 38

(iii) The adaptive immune response
17 Antigen recognition and processing 40
18 The antibody response 42
19 Antigen–antibody interaction and immune complexes 44
20 Cell-mediated immune responses 46

(iv) Regulation
21 Tolerance 48
22 Idiotypes, anti-idiotypes and networks 50
23 The cytokine network 52
24 Immunity, hormones and the brain 54

Potentially useful immunity
25 Anti-microbial immunity: a general scheme 56
26 Immunity to viruses 58
27 Immunity to bacteria 60
28 Immunity to fungi 62
29 Immunity to protozoa 64
30 Immunity to worms 66
31 Immunity to tumours 68

Undesirable effects of immunity
32 Harmful immunity: a general scheme 70
33 Allergy and anaphylaxis 72
34 Immune complexes, complement and disease 74
35 Chronic and cell-mediated inflammation 76
36 Autoimmunity 78
37 Transplant rejection 80

Altered immunity
38 Immunosuppression 82
39 Immunodeficiency 84
40 HIV and AIDS 86
41 Immunostimulation and vaccination 88

Appendices
42 Comparative sizes 90
   Comparative molecular weights 90
43 Landmarks in the history of immunology 91
   Some unsolved problems 91
44 The CD classification 92

Index 94

Preface

This is not a textbook for immunologists, who already have plenty of excellent volumes to choose from. Rather, it is aimed at all those on whose work immunology impinges but who may hitherto have lacked the time to keep abreast of a subject that can sometimes seem impossibly fast-moving and intricate.

Yet everyone with a background in medicine or the biological sciences is already familiar with a good deal of the basic knowledge required to understand immunological processes, often needing no more than a few quick blackboard sketches to see roughly how they work. This is a book of such sketches, which have proved useful over the years, recollected (and artistically touched up) in tranquillity.

The Chinese sage who remarked that one picture was worth a thousand words was certainly not an immunology teacher, or his estimate would not have been so low! In this book the text has been pruned to the minimum necessary for understanding the figures, omitting almost all historical and technical details, which can be found in the larger textbooks listed on the next page. In trying to steer a middle course between absolute clarity and absolute up-to-dateness, I am well aware of having missed both by a comfortable margin. But even in immunology, what is brand new does not always turn out to be right, while the idea that any form of presentation, however unorthodox, will make simple what other authors have already shown to be complex can only be, in Dr Johnson's heartfelt words, 'the dream of a philosopher doomed to wake a lexicographer'. My object has merely been to convince workers in neighbouring fields that modern immunology is not quite as forbidding as they may have thought.

It is perhaps the price of specialization that some important aspects of nature lie between disciplines and are consequently ignored for many years (transplant rejection is a good example). It follows that scientists are wise to keep an eye on each others' areas so that in due course the appropriate new disciplines can emerge—as immunology itself did from the shared interests of bacteriologists, haematologists, chemists, and the rest.

Acknowledgements

Our largest debt is obviously to the immunologists who made the discoveries this book is based on, if we had credited them all by name it would no longer have been a slim volume! In addition we are grateful to our colleagues at University College for advice and criticism since the first edition, particularly Professor J. Brostoff, Dr A. Cooke, Dr P. Delves, Dr V. Eisen, Professor F.C. Hay, Professor D.R. Katz, Dr T. Lund, Professor P.M. Lydyard, Dr D. Male, Dr S. Marshall-Clarke, Professor N.A. Mitchison, and Professor I.M. Roitt. The original draft was shown to Professor H.E.M. Kay, Professor C.A. Mims, and Professor L. Wolpert, all of whom made valuable suggestions. Edward Playfair supplied a useful undergraduate view. Finally we would like to thank the staff at Blackwell Science for help and encouragement at all stages.

Note on the seventh edition

Immunology never stands still, and since the sixth edition we have had to revise almost all sections of this book. The major changes will be found in the chapters on lymphocyte development, mucosal immunity, cytokines, tolerance, cell-mediated responses, and HIV/AIDS. We have updated the CD classification to the year 2000.

How to use this book

Each of the figures (listed in the contents) represents a particular topic, corresponding roughly to a 45-minute lecture. Newcomers to the subject may like first to read through the **text** (left-hand pages), using the figures only as a guide; this can be done at a sitting.

Once the general outline has been grasped, it is probably better to concentrate on the **figures** one at a time. Some of them are quite complicated and can certainly not be taken in 'at a glance', but will need to be worked through with the help of the **legends** (right-hand pages), consulting the **index** for further information on individual details; once this has been done carefully they should subsequently require little more than a cursory look to refresh the memory.

It will be evident that the figures are highly diagrammatic and not to scale; indeed the scale often changes several times within one figure. For an idea of the actual sizes of some of the cells and molecules mentioned, refer to **Appendix 1** (Section 42).

The reader will also notice that examples are drawn sometimes from the mouse, in which useful animal so much fundamental immunology has been worked out, and sometimes from the human, which is after all the one that matters to most people. Luckily the two species are, from the immunologist's viewpoint, remarkably similar.

Further reading

We cannot do better than recommend the textbooks we ourselves consult regularly, and which largely furnished the raw material for this book.

Abbas A.K., Lichtmann A.H. & Pober J.S. (1997) *Cellular and Molecular Immunology*. W.B. Saunders, Philadelphia (493 pp).

Austyn J.M. & Wood K.J. (1993) *Principles of Cellular and Molecular Immunology*. Oxford University Press, Oxford (735 pp).

Bibel D.J. (1988) *Milestones in Immunology*. Science-Tech Publishers, Madison, Wisconsin (330 pp).

Brostoff J., Scadding G.K., Male D. & Roitt I.M. (eds) (1991) *Clinical Immunology*. Mosby Europe, London (379 pp).

Goldsby R.A., Kindt T.J. & Osborne B.A. (2000) *Kuby Immunology*. 4th edn. W.H. Freeman, New York (650 pp).

Janeway C.A., Travers P., Walport M. & Capra J.D. (1999) *Immunology: the Immune System in Health and Disease*. 4th edn. Current Biology Limited, London (634 pp).

Lachmann P.J., Peters K., Rosen F.S. & Walport M.J. (eds) *Clinical Aspects of Immunology*. 5th edn. Blackwell Science, Oxford (2176 pp).

Mims C.A., Playfair J.H.L., Roitt I.M., Wakelin D. & Williams R. (1993) *Medical Microbiology*. Mosby, Europe (491 pp).

Peakman M. & Vergani D. (1997) *Basic and Clinical Immunology*. Churchill Livingstone, Edinburgh (338 pp).

Roitt I.M. (1997) *Essential Immunology*. 9th edn. Blackwell Science, Oxford (476 pp).

Roitt I.M., Brostoff J. & Male D. (1998) *Immunology*. 5th edn. Mosby, London (423 pp).

Roitt I.M. & Delves P.J. (eds) (1992) *Encyclopaedia of Immunology*. Academic Press, London (1578 pp).

Stites D., Terr A. & Parslow G. (eds) (1994) *Basic and Clinical Immunology*. 8th edn. Prentice-Hall, London (870 pp).

1 The scope of immunology

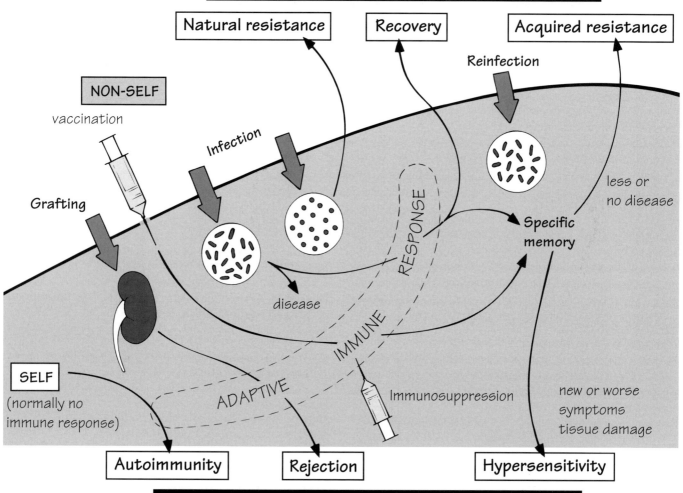

DESIRABLE CONSEQUENCES OF IMMUNITY

Natural resistance — Recovery — Acquired resistance

NON-SELF

vaccination

Grafting — Infection — Reinfection

less or no disease

disease

Specific memory

IMMUNE RESPONSE

ADAPTIVE

SELF (normally no immune response)

Immunosuppression

new or worse symptoms tissue damage

Autoimmunity — Rejection — Hypersensitivity

UNDESIRABLE CONSEQUENCES OF IMMUNITY

Of the four major causes of death—injury, infection, degenerative disease and cancer—only the first two regularly kill their victims before child-bearing age, which means that they are a potential source of lost genes. Therefore any mechanism that reduces their effects has tremendous survival value, and we see this in the processes, respectively, of **healing** and **immunity**.

Immunity is concerned with the recognition and disposal of foreign or 'non-self' material that enters the body (represented by grey arrows in the figure), usually in the form of life-threatening infectious micro-organisms but sometimes, unfortunately, in the shape of a life-saving kidney graft. Resistance to infection may be '**natural**' (i.e. inborn and unchanging) or '**acquired**' as the result of an **adaptive immune response** (centre).

Immunology is the study of the organs, cells, and molecules responsible for this recognition and disposal (the 'immune system'), of how they respond and interact, of the consequences—desirable (top) or otherwise (bottom)—of their activity, and of the ways in which they can be advantageously increased or reduced.

By far the most important type of foreign material that needs to be recognized and disposed of is the micro-organisms capable of causing infectious disease, and strictly speaking, immunity begins at the point when they enter the body. But it must be remembered that the first line of defence is to keep them out, and a variety of **external defences** have evolved for this purpose. Whether these are part of the immune system is a purely semantic question, but an immunologist is certainly expected to know about them.

Non-self A widely used term in immunology, covering everything which is detectably different from an animal's own constituents. Infectious micro-organisms, together with cells, organs, or other materials from another animal, are the most important non-self substances from an immunological viewpoint, but drugs and even normal foods which are, of course, non-self too, can sometimes give rise to immunity.

Infection Parasitic viruses, bacteria, protozoa, worms or fungi that attempt to gain access to the body or its surfaces are probably the chief *raison d'être* of the immune system. Higher animals whose immune system is damaged or deficient frequently succumb to infections which normal animals overcome.

External defences The presence of intact skin on the outside and mucous membranes lining the hollow viscera is in itself a powerful barrier against entry of potentially infectious organisms. In addition, there are numerous antimicrobial (mainly antibacterial) secretions in the skin and mucous surfaces. More specialized defences include the extreme acidity of the stomach (about pH2), and the mucus and upwardly beating cilia of the bronchial tree. Successful micro-organisms usually have cunning ways of breaching or evading these defences.

Natural resistance Organisms that enter the body (shown in the figure as black dots or rods) are often eliminated within minutes or hours by inborn, ever-present mechanisms, while others (the rods in the figure) can avoid this and survive, and may cause disease, unless they are dealt with by adaptive immunity (see below).

Adaptive immune response The development or augmentation of defence mechanisms in response to a particular ('specific') stimulus, e.g. an infectious organism. It can result in elimination of the micro-organism and **recovery** from disease, and often leaves the host with

specific memory, enabling it to respond more effectively on reinfection with the same micro-organism, a condition called **acquired resistance.** Since the body has no prior way of knowing which micro-organisms are harmless and which are not, all foreign material is usually responded to as if it were harmful, including relatively inoffensive pollens, etc.

Vaccination A method of stimulating the adaptive immune response and generating memory and acquired resistance without suffering the full effects of the disease. The name comes from *vaccinia*, or cowpox, used by Jenner to protect against smallpox.

Grafting Cells or organs from another individual usually survive natural resistance mechanisms but are attacked by the adaptive immune response, leading to **rejection**.

Autoimmunity The body's own ('self') cells and molecules do not normally stimulate its adaptive immune responses because of a variety of special mechanisms which ensure a state of **self-tolerance**, but in certain circumstances they do stimulate a response and the body's own structures are attacked as if they were foreign, a condition called **autoimmunity** or **autoimmune disease**.

Hypersensitivity Sometimes the result of specific memory is that re-exposure to the same stimulus, as well as or instead of eliminating the stimulus, has unpleasant or damaging effects on the body's own tissues. This is called **hypersensitivity**; examples are allergy (i.e. hay fever) and some forms of kidney disease. (Note, however, that the term 'allergy' is used by some immunologists to describe *all* alterations in responsiveness, in which case it also includes acquired resistance.)

Immunosuppression Autoimmunity, hypersensitivity, and above all graft rejection, sometimes necessitate the suppression of adaptive immune responses by drugs or other means.

2 Natural and adaptive immune mechanisms

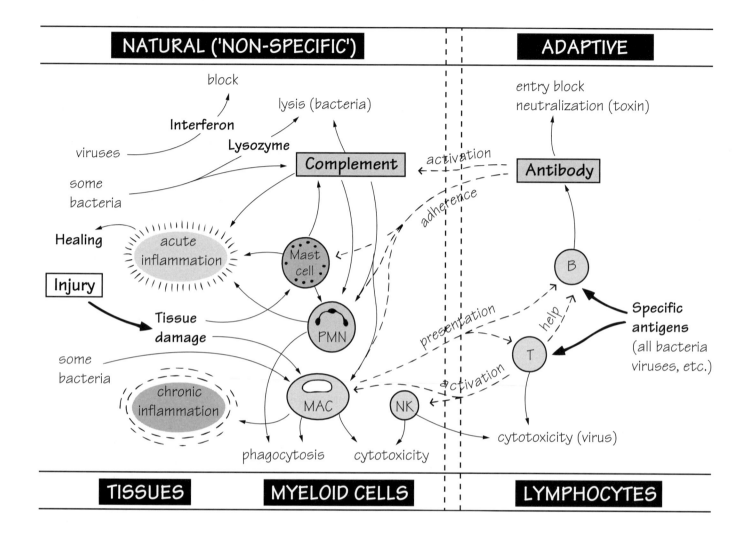

Just as resistance to disease can be natural (inborn) or acquired, the mechanisms mediating it can be correspondingly divided into **natural** (left) and **adaptive** (right), each composed of both **cellular** (lower) and **humoral** (i.e. free in serum or body fluids; upper half) elements. Adaptive mechanisms, more recently evolved, perform many of their functions by interacting with the older natural ones.

The mechanisms involved in natural immunity are largely the same as those responsible for non-specifically reacting to tissue damage, with the production of **inflammation** (cover up the right-hand part of the figure to appreciate this). However, some cells (e.g. macrophages) and some humoral factors (complement, lysozyme) do also have a limited ability to recognize and dispose of bacteria, while most cells can secrete interferon, which acts against viruses but not other types of organism. Thus the term 'non-specific', though often used as a synonym for 'natural', is not completely accurate.

Adaptive immunity is based on the special properties of **lymphocytes** (T and B, lower right), which can respond selectively to thousands of different non-self materials, or 'antigens', leading to specific memory and a permanently altered pattern of response—an *adaptation* to the animal's own surroundings. Adaptive mechanisms can function on their own against certain antigens (cover up the left-hand part of the figure), but the majority of their effects are exerted by means of the interaction of antibody with complement and the phagocytic cells of natural immunity, and of T cells with macrophages (broken lines). Through their activation of these natural mechanisms, adaptive responses frequently provoke **inflammation**, either acute or chronic; when it becomes a nuisance this is called **hypersensitivity**.

The individual elements of this highly simplified scheme are illustrated in more detail in the remainder of this book.

Natural immunity

Interferon A family of proteins produced rapidly by many cells in response to virus infection, which block the replication of virus in other cells. Interferons also play an important role in communication between immune cells (see Fig. 23).

Lysozyme (muramidase) An enzyme secreted by macrophages, which attacks the cell wall of some bacteria. Interferon and lysozyme are sometimes described as 'natural antibiotics'.

Complement A series of enzymes present in serum which when activated produce widespread inflammatory effects, as well as lysis of bacteria, etc. Some bacteria activate complement directly, while others only do so with the help of antibody (see Fig. 5).

Lysis Irreversible leakage of cell contents following membrane damage. In the case of a bacterium this would be fatal to the microbe.

Mast cell A large tissue cell which releases inflammatory mediators when damaged, and also under the influence of antibody. By increasing vascular permeability, inflammation allows complement and cells to enter the tissues from the blood (see Fig. 6 for further details of this process).

PMN Polymorphonuclear leucocyte, a short-lived 'scavenger' blood cell, whose granules contain powerful bactericidal enzymes.

MAC Macrophage, a large tissue cell responsible for removing damaged tissue, cells, bacteria, etc. Both PMNs and macrophages come from the bone marrow, and are therefore known as **myeloid** cells.

Dendritic cells A rare cell type found in the T cell area of all lymphoid tissues, whose function is to present antigen to T cells, and thus initiate all T cell-dependent immune responses. Not to be confused with follicular dendritic cells, which store antigen for B cells (see Fig. 18).

Phagocytosis ('cell eating') Engulfment of a particle by a cell. Macrophages and PMNs (which used to be called 'microphages') are the most important phagocytic cells. The great majority of foreign materials entering the tissues are ultimately disposed of by this mechanism.

Cytotoxicity Macrophages can kill some targets (perhaps including tumour cells) without phagocytosing them, and there are a variety of other cells with cytotoxic abilities.

NK (natural killer) cell A lymphocyte-like cell capable of killing some targets, notably virus-infected cells and tumour cells, but without the receptor or the fine specificity characteristic of true lymphocytes.

Adaptive immunity

Antigen Strictly speaking, a substance which stimulates the production of **antibody**. The term is often applied, however, to substances that stimulate any type of adaptive immune response. Typically, antigens are foreign ('non-self') and either particulate (e.g. cells, bacteria, etc.) or large protein or polysaccharide molecules. But under special conditions small molecules and even 'self' components can become antigenic. The principal requirement of an antigen is some surface feature detectably foreign to the animal, though there is more to it than this (see Figs 17–20).

Specific; specificity Terms used to denote the production of an immune response more or less selective for the stimulus, such as a lymphocyte which responds to, or an antibody which 'fits', a particular antigen. For example, antibody against measles virus will not bind to mumps virus: it is 'specific' for measles.

Lymphocyte A small cell found in blood, from which it recirculates through the tissues and back via the lymph, 'policing' the body for non-self material. Its ability to recognize individual antigens through its specialized surface receptors and to divide into numerous cells of identical specificity and long lifespan, makes it the ideal cell for adaptive responses. Two major populations of lymphocytes are recognized: T and B (see also Fig. 9).

B lymphocytes secrete antibody, the humoral element of adaptive immunity.

T ('thymus-derived') lymphocytes are further divided into subpopulations which 'help' B lymphocytes, kill virus-infected cells, activate macrophages, etc.

Interactions between natural and adaptive immunity

Antibody Serum globulins with a wide range of specificity for different antigens. Although antibodies can bind to and neutralize bacterial toxins directly, they exert most of their effect by binding to the surface of bacteria, viruses, or other parasites, and thus increasing their adherence to, and phagocytosis by, myeloid cells. This phenomenon is known as opsonization. Antibody also activates complement on the surface of invading pathogens.

Complement As mentioned above, complement is often activated by antibody bound to microbial surfaces. However, binding of complement to antigen can also greatly increase its ability to activate a strong and lasting B cell response—an example of 'reverse interaction' between adaptive and natural immune mechanisms.

Presentation of antigens to T and B cells by dendritic cells is necessary for most adaptive responses; presentation by dendritic cells usually requires activation of these cells by elements of the 'natural' immune system, another example of 'reverse interaction' between adaptive and natural immune mechanisms.

Help by T cells is required for many branches of the immune response. T cell help is required for the secretion of most antibodies by B cells and for activating macrophages to stimulate cellular immunity. T cell help is also required for an effective cytotoxic T cell response. There are also 'suppressor' or 'regulator' T cells which have the opposite effect.

3 Evolution of immune mechanisms

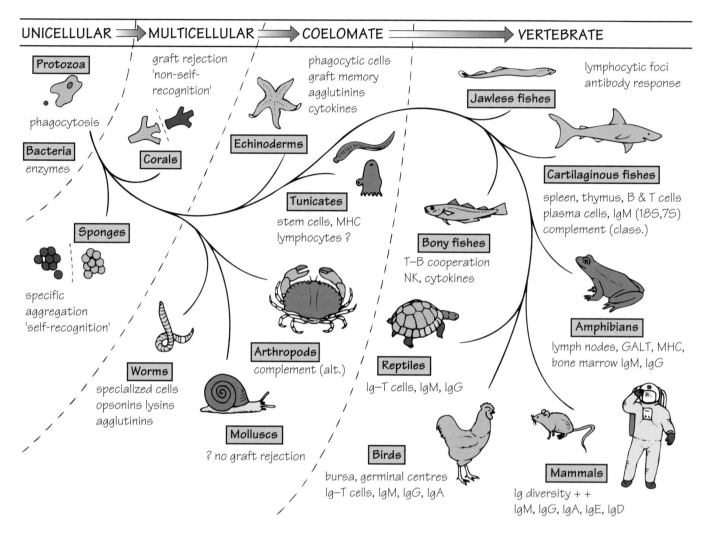

UNICELLULAR ⟹ MULTICELLULAR ⟹ COELOMATE ⟹ VERTEBRATE

Protozoa

phagocytosis

Bacteria
enzymes

graft rejection
'non-self-
recognition'

Corals

Echinoderms

phagocytic cells
graft memory
agglutinins
cytokines

Tunicates
stem cells, MHC
lymphocytes ?

Sponges

specific
aggregation
'self-recognition'

Worms
specialized cells
opsonins lysins
agglutinins

Arthropods
complement (alt.)

Molluscs
? no graft rejection

Bony fishes
T–B cooperation
NK, cytokines

Reptiles
Ig–T cells, IgM, IgG

Birds
bursa, germinal centres
Ig–T cells, IgM, IgG, IgA

Jawless fishes

lymphocytic foci
antibody response

Cartilaginous fishes
spleen, thymus, B & T cells
plasma cells, IgM (18S,7S)
complement (class.)

Amphibians
lymph nodes, GALT, MHC,
bone marrow IgM, IgG

Mammals
Ig diversity + +
IgM, IgG, IgA, IgE, IgD

From the humble amoeba searching for food (top left) to the mammal with its sophisticated humoral and cellular immune mechanisms (bottom right), the process of '**self vs. non-self recognition**' shows a steady development, keeping pace with the increasing need of animals to maintain their integrity in a hostile environment. The decision at which point 'immunity' appeared is thus a purely semantic one.

In this figure some of the important landmarks in this development are shown. Since most advances, once achieved, persist in subsequent species, they have for clarity been shown only where they are first thought to have appeared. It must be remembered that our knowledge of primitive animals is based largely on study of their modern descendants, all of whom evidently have immune systems adequate to their circumstances.

In so far as the T cell system is based on the cellular recognition of 'altered-self' or 'not-quite-self', it appears to have its roots considerably further back in evolution than antibody, which is roughly restricted to vertebrates. In mammals we can distinguish three separate **recognition systems**, based on molecules expressed on B cells only (antibody), on T cells only (the T cell receptor), and on a range of cells (the major histo-

compatibility complex, MHC), all of which look as if their genes evolved from a single primitive precursor (see Fig. 12 for further details). In addition, recent studies have indicated that vertebrates share with insects (and perhaps other invertebrates) recognition systems which respond to common molecular patterns found on the surface of microbes (e.g. lipopolysaccharides).

Lymphocytes, with their characteristic properties of **specificity** and **memory**, appear not to have evolved until the earliest vertebrates, which gives rise to the common generalization that adaptive immunity is restricted to vertebrates. Why this should be has never been totally explained, but one can imagine that vertebrate existence brought with it a variety of increases that would put extra demands on immune defences against infection—e.g. size, lifespan, body temperature, choice of habitat—but the real link between backbones and lymphocytes is not obvious and with the improvement of techniques for studying the DNA of early animals and even fossils, plenty of surprises can still be expected. Moreover the existence of immune mechanisms in plants is only now beginning to be systematically explored.

Invertebrates

Protozoa Lacking chlorophyll, these little animals must eat. Little is known about how they recognize 'food', but their surface proteins are under quite complex genetic control.

Bacteria We think of bacteria as parasites, but they themselves can suffer from infection by specialized viruses called bacteriophages. It is thought that the restriction endonucleases, so indispensable to the modern genetic engineer, have as their real function the recognition and destruction of viral DNA without damage to that of the host bacterium. Successful bacteriophages have evolved resistance to this, a beautiful example of natural immunity and its limitations.

Sponges Partly free-living, partly colonial, sponge cells use species-specific glycoproteins to identify 'self' and prevent hybrid colony formation. If forced together, non-identical colonies undergo necrosis at the contact zone, with accelerated breakdown of a second graft.

Corals Corals accept genetically identical grafts (syngrafts) but slowly reject non-identical ones (allografts) with damage to both partners. There is some evidence for specific memory of a previous rejection—i.e. of 'adaptive' immunity.

Worms A feature of all coelomate animals is cell specialization. In the earthworm coelom there are at least four cell types, some of which are involved in allograft rejection, while others may produce antibacterial factors; all are phagocytic.

Molluscs and **arthropods** are curious in apparently not showing graft rejection. However, humoral factors are prominent, possibly including the earliest complement (alternative pathway) components, which may be responsible for their resistance to some parasites. Insect immune systems have been studied in most detail, and families of receptors ('toll' receptors) have been described which trigger the synthesis of antimicrobial proteins in response to molecular structures found on the surface of insect pathogens (e.g. some polysaccharides on the surface of fungi).

Echinoderms The starfish is famous for Metchnikoff's classic demonstration of specialized phagocytic cells in 1882. Allografts are rejected, with cellular infiltration, and there is a strong specific memory response. Molecules resembling the cytokines IL-1 (interleukin-1) and TNF (tumour necrosis factor) have been identified in these and other invertebrates.

Tunicates (e.g. *Amphioxus*, sea-squirts) These prevertebrates show several advanced features; self-renewing haemopoietic cells, lymphoid-like cells, and a single MHC controlling the rejection of foreign grafts.

Vertebrates

Jawless fishes (cyclostomes, e.g. hagfish, lamprey) The earliest surviving vertebrates, with lymphoid cells organized into foci in the pharynx and elsewhere, and the first definite antibody immunoglobulin (Ig), a labile four-chain molecule, produced specifically in response to a variety of antigens: a dramatic moment in the evolution of the immune system. Note that other molecules of the 'immunoglobulin superfamily', for example adhesion molecules, are already present in invertebrates such as the arthropods.

Cartilaginous fishes (e.g. sharks) The first appearance of the thymus, of the secondary antibody response, and of plasma cells (specialized for high-rate antibody secretion) marks another tremendous step. Ig chains are now disulphide-linked; the high and low molecular weight forms probably represent polymerization rather than class differences. Molecules of the classical complement pathway also make their appearance.

Bony fish The different responses to mitogens and the evidence for cell Cupertino in antibody production suggest that T and B lymphocyte functions have begun to separate and there is evidence for NK cells and cytokines (e.g. IL-2, IFN) at least as early as this. Zebra fishes appear to contain a polymorphic MHC system similar to that of mammals.

Amphibians The first appearance of another Ig class (IgG) (see Fig. 16) and of clear-cut MHC antigens. During morphogenesis (e.g. tadpole → frog) specific tolerance may develop towards the new antigens of the adult stage. Lymph nodes and gut-associated lymphoid tissue (GALT) and haemopoiesis in the bone marrow also appear for the first time.

Reptiles were previously thought to carry on their thymus cells Ig similar to that in serum, but the probability is that this is in fact the antecedent of the T cell receptor and that the antisera used for its detection 'cross-reacted' with Ig—a common problem in immunology.

Birds are unusual in producing their B lymphocytes exclusively in a special organ, the bursa of Fabricius, near the cloaca. They have a large multilobular thymus but no conventional lymph nodes. Their complement system is also very different from that of mammals; for example Factor B appears to take the place of C4 and C2 (see Fig. 5).

Mammals are characterized more by diversity of Ig classes and subclasses, and MHC antigens, than by any further development of effector functions. There are some curious variations; for example rats have unusually strong natural immunity and some animals (whales, Syrian hamsters) show surprisingly little MHC polymorphism. However, humans and mice, fortunately (for the humans), are immunologically remarkably similar.

4 Cells involved in immunity: the haemopoietic system

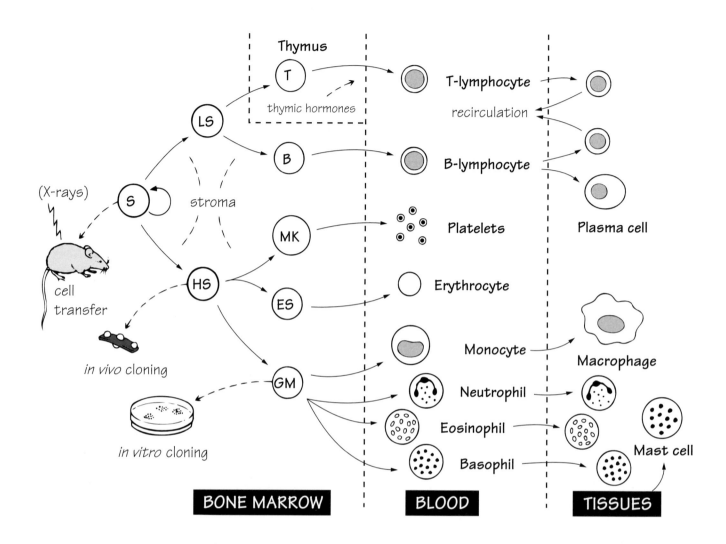

The great majority of cells involved in mammalian immunity are derived from precursors in the **bone marrow** (left half of figure) and circulate in the **blood**, entering and sometimes leaving the **tissues** when required.

The existence of the long-debated totipotent **stem cell** in the adult, retaining the 'embryonic' ability to differentiate into all types of blood cell, has been established by cell-transfer experiments and chromosome analysis in irradiated mice (centre left); stem cells are probably restricted to the bone marrow and blood and are very rare there (about one in 100 000 cells). By injecting small numbers of marrow cells, discrete spleen nodules, or 'in vivo' clones can be grown, whose morphology and differentiation can be studied in a more or less natural environment. Similar experiments in semisolid culture conditions *in vitro*

enable the clonal progeny of single marrow cells to be examined in complete isolation (lower left). Based on this approach, haematologists use a complex terminology of 'colony-forming' and 'burst-forming units' (CFU, BFU). Proliferation and differentiation of all these cells is under the control of **growth factors** released by the bone marrow stroma and by each other (see Fig. 23).

Unlike other haemopoietic cells, lymphocytes do not normally divide unless stimulated, and the propagation of lymphocyte clones usually requires repeated exposure to antigen and growth factors, followed by selection of specifically reactive cells. But T or B lymphocytes can be fused with a tumour cell, to produce an immortal hybrid clone or 'hybridoma', of great value in studying the properties of lymphocytes, which are complex and varied (see Fig. 9).

A note on terminology

Haematologists recognize many stages between stem cells and their fully differentiated progeny (e.g. for the red cells: proerythroblast; erythroblast, normoblast, erythrocyte). The suffix **blast** usually implies an early, dividing, relatively undifferentiated cell, but is also used to describe lymphocytes that have been stimulated, e.g. by antigen, and are about to divide; whence the term 'blast transformation'.

Stroma Endothelial and other non-haemopoietic cells that provide support and secrete growth factors for haemopoiesis.

S Stem cell; the totipotent and self-renewing marrow cell, of proved existence but uncertain morphology. Stem cells are found in low numbers in blood as well as bone marrow and the numbers can be boosted by treatment with appropriate growth factors (e.g. G-CSF). This has important clinical implications, since it greatly facilitates the process of 'bone marrow' transplantation (see Fig. 37).

LS Lymphoid stem cell, presumed to be capable of differentiating into T or B lymphocytes.

HS Haemopoietic stem cell; the precursor of spleen nodules and probably able to differentiate into all but the lymphoid pathways—granulocyte, erythroid, monocyte, megakaryocyte; often referred to as CFU-GEMM.

ES Erythroid stem cell, destined to differentiate into erythrocytes. Haematologists distinguish the BFU and the later CFU on the basis of their growth patterns *in vitro*. As well as the locally produced growth factors (see below), erythropoietin, a glycoprotein hormone formed in the kidney in response to hypoxia, accelerates the differentiation of red cell precursors and thus adjusts the production of red cells to the demand for their oxygen-carrying capacity—a typical example of 'negative feedback'.

GM or CFU G/M Granulocyte–monocyte common precursor; a cell capable of differentiating into various cells of the myeloid series depending on the presence of 'growth-' or 'colony-stimulating' factors.

Neutrophil (polymorph) The commonest leucocyte of the blood, a short-lived phagocytic cell whose granules contain numerous bactericidal substances.

Eosinophil A leucocyte whose large refractile granules contain a number of highly basic or 'cationic' proteins, possibly important in killing larger parasites including worms.

Basophil A leucocyte whose large basophilic granules contain heparin and vasoactive amines, important in the inflammatory response.

The above three cell types are often collectively referred to as 'granulocytes.'

MK Megakaryocyte; the parent cell of the blood platelets.

Platelets Small cells responsible for sealing damaged blood vessels ('haemostasis') but also the source of many inflammatory mediators (see Fig. 6).

Monocyte The largest nucleated cell of the blood, developing into a macrophage when it migrates into the tissues.

Macrophage The principal resident phagocyte of the tissues and serous cavities such as the pleura and peritoneum.

Dendritic cell Rare cell type whose function is to present antigens to T cells. In lymphoid tissue these cells show characteristic long dendritic processes which enable them to interact with many T cells at the same time. Precursors of these cells are found in all tissues of the body (e.g. the Langerhans' cells of the skin) where they take up antigen and then migrate to the T cell areas of the lymph node or spleen via the lymphatics or the blood.

T Thymus-derived (or -processed) lymphocyte.

Thymic hormones Numerous small peptides extracted from thymic epithelium (e.g. 'thymosin') are thought by some to assist the differentiation of T lymphocytes (see Figs 9–11 for further details of lymphocyte development).

B Bone marrow-(or, in birds, bursa-) derived lymphocyte, the precursor of antibody-forming cells. In fetal life, the liver may play the role of 'bursa'.

Plasma cell A B cell in its high-rate antibody-secreting state. Despite their name, plasma cells are seldom seen in the blood, but are found in spleen, lymph nodes, etc., whenever antibody is being made.

Mast cell A large tissue cell similar in appearance and function to the basophil, but thought not to originate from the bone marrow. Mast cells are easily triggered by tissue damage to initiate the inflammatory response. (See Fig. 33 for details of mast cell subpopulations.)

Growth factors With the exception of erythropoietin and the thymic hormones (see above), the molecules that control the proliferation and differentiation of haemopoietic cells are the same as those involved in many immune responses—the interleukins (see Fig. 23)—but some of them were first discovered by haematologists and are called 'colony-stimulating factors' (CSF). The different names have no real significance, indeed one interleukin, IL-3, is often known as 'multi-CSF'. Growth factors are used in clinical practice to boost particular subsets of blood cell, and erythropoetin was in fact one of the first of the new generation of proteins produced by 'recombinant' technology to be used in the clinic.

5 Complement

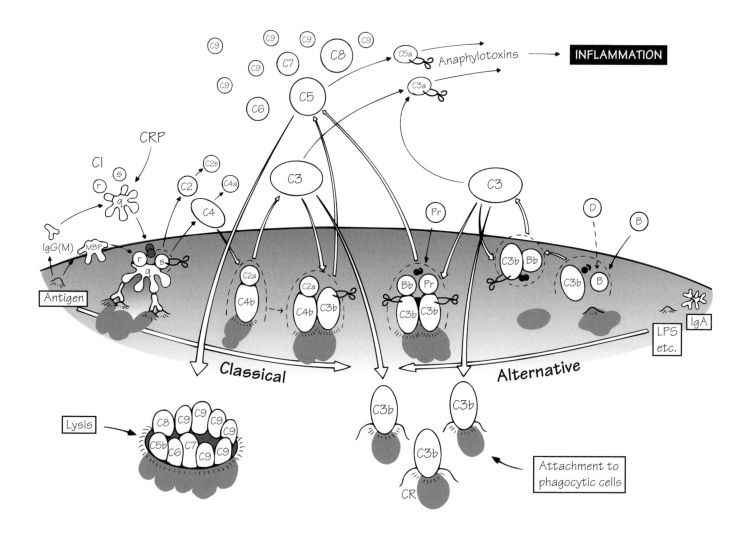

Fifteen or more serum components constitute the **complement** system, whose sequential activation and assembly into functional units leads to three main effects: release of peptides active in **inflammation** (top right), deposition of C3b, a powerful attachment-promoter (or 'opsonin') for **phagocytosis**, on cell membranes (bottom right), and membrane damage resulting in **lysis** (bottom left). Together these make it an important part of the defences against micro-organisms. Defects of some components can predispose to severe infections, particularly bacterial (see Fig. 39).

The upper half of the figure represents the serum, or 'fluid' phase, the lower half the cell surface, where activation (indicated by dotted haloes) and assembly largely occur. Activation of complement can proceed by two distinct routes, the '**classical**' (because first described) pathway, initiated by the binding of specific antibody of the IgG or IgM class (see Fig. 16) to surface antigens (centre left), and the '**alternative**', but probably more primitive, pathway, initiated by a variety of polysaccharides and by

some antibodies (centre right). Some of the steps are dependent on the divalent ions Ca^{2+} (shaded circles) or Mg^{2+} (black circles). A key feature of complement function is that it functions via a biochemical **cascade**: a single activation event (whether by antibody or via the alternative pathway) leading to the production of many down-stream events, such as deposition of C3b.

Activation is usually limited to the immediate vicinity by the very short life of the active products, and in some cases there are special inactivators ( ). Nevertheless, excessive complement activation can cause unpleasant side-effects (see Fig. 34).

Note that in the absence of antibody, many of the molecules that activate the complement system are carbohydrate or lipid in nature, for example lipopolysaccharides, mannose, suggesting that the system evolved mainly to recognize bacterial surfaces via their non-protein features. With the appearance of antibody in the vertebrates (see Fig. 3) it became possible for virtually any foreign molecule to activate the system.

Classical pathway

For many years this was the only way in which complement was known to be activated. The essential feature is the requirement for a specific antigen–antibody interaction, leading via components C1, C2 and C4 to the formation of a 'convertase' which splits C3.

MBP Mannose-binding protein, a C1q-like molecule that recognizes microbial components such as yeast mannan and activates C1r and s.

CRP C-reactive protein, produced in large amounts during 'acute-phase' responses (see Fig. 6), binds to bacterial phosphoryl choline and activates C1q.

Ig IgM and some subclasses of IgG (in the human, IgG3, 1 and 2), when bound to antigen are recognized by C1q to initiate the classical pathway.

C1 A Ca^{2+} dependent union of three components: C1q (MW 400 000), a curious protein with six valencies for Ig linked by collagen-like fibrils, which activates in turn C1r (MW 170 000) and C1s (MW 80 000), a serine esterase which goes on to attack C2 and C4.

C2 (MW 120 000), split by C1s into small (C2b) and large (C2a) fragments.

C4 (MW 240 000), likewise split into C4a (small) and C4b (large). C4b and C2a then join together and attach to the antigen–antibody complex, or to the membrane in the case of a cell-bound antigen, forming a 'C3 convertase'. Note that some complementologists prefer to reverse the names of C2a and b, so that for both C2 and C4 the 'a' peptide is the smaller one.

C3 (MW 180 000), the central component of all complement reactions, split by its convertase into a small (C3a) and a large fragment (C3b). Some of the C3b is deposited on the membrane, where it serves as an attachment site for phagocytic polymorphs and macrophages, which have receptors for it; some remains associated with C2a and C4b, forming a 'C5 convertase'. Two 'C3b inactivator' enzymes rapidly inactivate C3b, releasing the fragment C3c and leaving membrane-bound C3d.

C5 (MW 180 000), split by its convertase into C5a, a small peptide which, together with C3a (anaphylotoxins), acts on mast cells, polymorphs and smooth muscle to promote the inflammatory response, and C5b, which initiates the assembly of C6, 7, 8 and 9 into the membrane-damaging or 'lytic' unit.

CR Complement receptor. Three types of molecule that bind different products of C3 breakdown are found on cell surfaces: CR1 on red cells, CR1 and CR3 on phagocytic cells, where they act as opsonins (see Fig. 8) and CR2 on B lymphocytes where it may be involved in the induction of memory but is also, unfortunately, the receptor via which the Epstein–Barr virus gains entry (see Fig. 26).

Alternative pathway

The principal features distinguishing this from the classical pathway are the lack of dependence on calcium ions and the lack of need for C1, C2 or C4, and therefore for specific antigen–antibody interaction. Instead, several different molecules can initiate C3 conversion, notably lipopolysaccharides (LPS) and other bacterial products, but also including aggregates of some types of antibody such as IgA (see Fig. 16). Essentially the alternative pathway consists of a continuously 'ticking over' cycle, held in check by control molecules whose effects are counteracted by the various initiators.

B Factor B (MW 100 000), which complexes with C3b, whether produced via the classical pathway or the alternative pathway itself. It has both structural and functional similarities to C2, and both are coded for by genes within the very important major histocompatibility complex (see Fig. 13). In birds, which lack C2 and C4, C1 activates Factor B.

D Factor D (MW 25 000), an enzyme which acts on the C3b–B complex to produce the active convertase, referred to in the language of complementologists as C3bBb.

Pr Properdin (MW 220 000), the first isolated component of the alternative pathway, once thought to be the actual initiator but now known merely to stabilize the C3b–B complex so that it can act on further C3. Thus more C3b is produced which, with Factors B and D, leads in turn to further C3 conversion—a 'positive feedback' loop with great amplifying potential (but restrained by the C3b inactivators Factor H and Factor I).

Lytic pathway

Lysis of cells is probably the least vital of the complement reactions, but one of the easiest to study. It is initiated by the splitting of C5 by one of its two convertases: C3b–C2a–C4b (classical pathway) or C3b–Bb–Pr (alternative pathway). Thereafter the results are the same, however caused.

C6 (MW 150 000), **C7** (MW 140 000) and **C8** (MW 150 000) unite with C5b, one molecule of each, and with 10 or more molecules of **C9** (MW 80 000). This 'membrane attack complex' is shaped somewhat like a cylindrical tube and when inserted into the membrane of bacteria, red cells, etc. causes leakage of the contents and death or lysis. Needless to say, bacteria have evolved various strategies for avoiding this (see Fig. 27).

Complement inhibitors

In order to prevent over-activation of the complement cascade, there are numerous inhibitory mechanisms regulating complement. Some of these, like C1q inhibitor, block the activity of complement proteinases. Others cleave active complement components into inactive fragments (factor I). Yet others destabilize the molecular complexes which build up during complement activation. Genetic manipulation has been used to make pigs carrying a transgene coding for the human version of one such important regulatory protein DAF (decay accelerating factor); results suggest that tissues from such pigs are less rapidly rejected when transplanted into primates, increasing the chances of carrying out successful xenotransplanation (see Fig. 37).

6 Acute inflammation

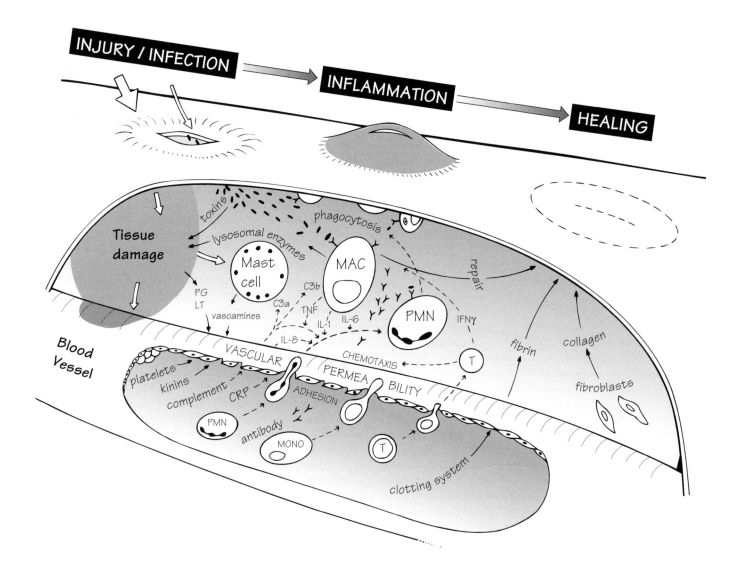

Whether **inflammation** should be considered part of immunology is a problem for the teaching profession, not for the body—which combats infection by all the means at its disposal, including mechanisms also involved in the response to and repair of other types of damage.

In this simplified scheme, which should be read from left to right, are shown the effects of **injury** to tissues (top left) and to blood vessels (bottom left). The small black rods represent bacterial **infection**, a very common cause of inflammation and of course a frequent accompaniment of injury. Note the central role of **permeability of the vascular endothelium** in allowing access of blood cells and serum components (lower half) to the tissues (upper half), which also accounts for the main symptoms of inflammation—redness, warmth, swelling and pain.

It can be seen that the 'adaptive' (or 'immunological') functions of antibody and lymphocytes largely operate to amplify or focus pre-existing 'natural' mechanisms; quantitatively, however, they are so important that they frequently make the difference between life and death. Further details of the role of antibody and lymphocytes in inflammation can be found in Figs 32–36.

Note the central importance of the tissue **mast cells** and **macrophages**, and the blood-derived **PMN**. If for any reason inflammation does not die down within a matter of days, it may become chronic, and here the macrophage and the T lymphocyte play dominant roles (see Fig. 35).

Mast cell A large tissue cell with basophilic granules containing vasoactive amines and heparin. It degranulates readily in response to injury by trauma, heat, UV light, etc. and also in some allergic conditions (see Fig. 33).

PG, LT Prostaglandins and leukotrienes; a family of unsaturated fatty acids (MW 300–400) derived by metabolism of arachidonic acid, a component of most cell membranes. Individual PGs and LTs have different but overlapping effects; together they are responsible for the induction of pain, fever, vascular permeability and chemotaxis of PMN, and some of them also inhibit lymphocyte functions.

Vasoamines Vasoactive amines; for example, histamine, 5-hydroxy-tryptamine, produced by mast cells, basophils and platelets, and causing increased capillary permeability.

Kinin system A series of serum peptides sequentially activated to cause vasodilation and increased permeability.

Complement A cascading sequence of serum proteins, activated either directly ('alternate pathway') or via antigen–antibody interaction (see Fig. 5 for details of the individual components).

C3a and C5a which stimulate release by mast cells of their vasoactive amines, are known as anaphylotoxins.

Opsonization C3b attached to a particle promotes sticking to phagocytic cells because of their 'C3 receptors'. Antibody, if present, augments this by binding to 'Fc receptors'.

CRP C-reactive protein (MW 130000), a pentameric globulin made in the liver which appears in the serum within hours of tissue damage or infection, and whose ancestry goes back to the invertebrates. It binds to phosphorylcholine, which is found on the surface of many bacteria, fixes complement and promotes phagocytosis, thus it may play an antibody-like role in some bacterial infections. Proteins whose serum concentration increases during inflammation are called 'acute phase proteins'; they include CRP and many complement components, as well as other microbe-binding molecules and enzyme inhibitors. This **acute phase response** can be viewed as a rapid, not very specific, attempt to deal with more or less any type of infection or damage.

PMN Polymorphonuclear leucocyte; the major mobile phagocytic cell, whose prompt arrival in the tissues plays a vital part in removing invading bacteria.

Mono Monocyte; the precursor of tissue macrophages (MAC in the figure) which is responsible for removing damaged tissue as well as micro-organisms. The tissue macrophages are also an important source of the inflammatory cytokines TNF-α, IL-1, and IL-6 (see below).

Lysosomal enzymes Bactericidal enzymes released from the lysosomes of PMNs, monocytes and macrophages, e.g. lysozyme, myeloperoxidase and others, also capable of damaging normal tissues.

Inflammatory cytokines The inflammatory response is orchestrated by several cytokines, which are produced by a variety of cell types. The most important are TNF-α, IL-6 and IL-1. All these cytokines have many functions (they are 'pleiotropic'), including initiating many of the changes in the vascular endothelium which promote leucocyte entry into the inflammatory site. They also induce the acute phase response and, later, the process of tissue repair. IL-1 is one of the few cytokines which act systemically, rather than locally—for example, through its action on the hypothalamus, it is the main molecule responsible for inducing fever. See Fig. 23 for further details of cytokines.

Chemotaxis C5a, C3a, leukotrienes and 'chemokines' stimulate PMNs and monocytes to move into the tissues. Movement towards the site of inflammation is called chemotaxis, and is presumably due to the cells' ability to detect a concentration gradient of chemotactic factors; random increases of movement are called chemokinesis.

Chemokines These are a very large family of small polypeptides, which play a key role in chemotaxis and the regulation of leucocyte trafficking. There are three main classes of chemokines (α, β and γ) based on the distribution of conserved disulphide bonds. They bind to an equally large family of chemokine receptors, and the biology of the system is further complicated by the fact that many of the chemokines have multiple functions, and can bind to many different receptors. Although some have been called interleukins (e.g. IL 8), the majority have retained separate names. They shot to prominence when it was discovered that some of the chemokine receptors (e.g. the CCR5 receptor) served as essential coreceptors (together with CD4) for HIV to gain entry into cells (see Fig. 40).

Adhesion and cell traffic Changes in the expression of endothelial surface molecules, induced mainly by cytokines, cause PMN, monocytes, and lymphocytes to slow down and subsequently adhere to the vessel wall. These 'adhesion molecules' and the molecules they bind to fall into well-defined groups (selectins, integrins, the Ig superfamily, see Fig. 12). These changes, together with the selective local release of **chemokines**, regulate the changes in cell traffic which underlie all inflammatory responses.

T T lymphocyte, undergoing **blast** transformation if stimulated by antigen, as is the case in most infections. By releasing cytokines such as IFNγ (see Fig. 23), T cells can greatly increase the activity of macrophages.

Clotting system Intimately bound up with complement and kinins because of several shared activation steps. Blood clotting is a vital part of the healing process.

Fibrin The end product of blood clotting and, in the tissues, the matrix into which fibroblasts migrate to initiate healing.

Fibroblast An important tissue cell which migrates into the fibrin clot and secretes **collagen**, an enormously strong polymerizing molecule giving the healing wound its strength and elasticity. Subsequently new blood capillaries sprout into the area, leading eventually to the restoration of the normal architecture.

7 Phagocytic cells: the reticulo-endothelial system

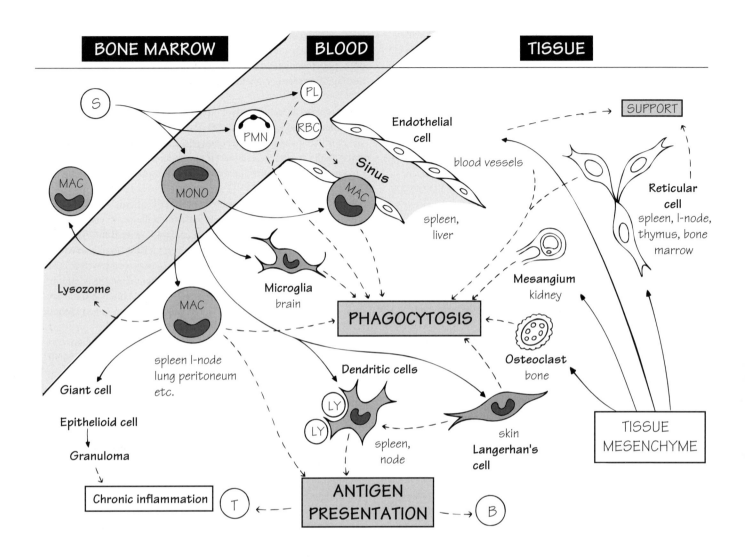

Particulate matter which finds its way into the blood or tissues is rapidly removed by cells, and the property of taking up dyes, colloids, etc., was used by anatomists to define a body-wide system of **phagocytic** cells known as the '**reticulo-endothelial system**' (RES), consisting of the vascular endothelium and reticular tissue cells (top right), and—supposedly descended from these—various types of macrophages whose routine functions included clearing up the body's own debris and killing and digesting bacteria.

However, more modern work has shown a fundamental distinction between those phagocytic cells derived from the bone marrow via the blood monocyte (shaded) and others formed locally from the tissues themselves (right side of figure). Ironically, neither reticular nor endothelial cells are outstandingly phagocytic. Their function is partly structural, in maintaining the integrity of the lymphoid tissue and blood vessels, respectively. However, there is increasing awareness that both cell types have an equally important role, as 'signposts' regulating the migration of haemopoetic cells from blood into the tissues and through the various subcompartments of lymphoid tissue. In contrast, the major phagocytic tissue cell is the macrophage, and it is therefore more usual today to speak of the '**mononuclear phagocytic system**' (MPS).

More recently still, attention has focused on the interactions between the RES and adaptive immunity. The role of antibody in amplifying phagocytosis and of T lymphocytes in activating other macrophage functions is discussed in Figs 8 and 35, but it is worth noting here that neither B nor T lymphocytes can normally respond to foreign antigens unless the latter are properly '**presented**'. It used to be assumed that the presenting cells were typical macrophages, but it is now clear that there are special separate populations of cells in the skin and the lymphoid organs (lower centre) with the ability to bind protein antigens and break them down into small peptides, which associate with MHC molecules and are then recognized by T cells (see Fig. 17).

Endothelial cell   The inner lining of blood vessels, able to take up dyes, etc., but not truly phagocytic. There is, however, evidence that endothelial cells can present antigen to lymphocytes under some circumstances, and they can both produce and respond to cytokines rather as macrophages do.

Reticular cell   The main supporting or 'stromal' cell of lymphoid organs, usually associated with the collagen-like reticulin fibres, and not easily distinguished from fibroblasts or from other branching or 'dendritic' cells (see below)—whence a great deal of confusion.

Mesangium   Mesangial cells give support to the glomerulus, and may phagocytose material deposited in it, particularly complexes of antigen and antibody.

Osteoclast   A large multinucleate cell responsible for resorbing and so shaping bone. There is some evidence that its function can be regulated by T lymphocytes.

Dendritic cells   The weakly phagocytic **Langerhans cell** of the epidermis, and somewhat similar but non-phagocytic cells in the lymphoid follicles of the spleen and lymph nodes, are the main agents of T cell stimulation; T cells recognize foreign antigens in association with cell-surface antigens coded for by the MHC, a genetic region intimately involved in immune responses of all kinds (see Figs 13, 14, 17, 20). There are separate follicular dendritic cells for presenting antigen to B cells which specialize in trapping antigen-antibody complexes. All cells of this type appear to be derived from the bone marrow. The 'veiled' cells seen in the lymph are thought to be Langerhans cells bearing antigen, en route to the lymph node where they become interdigitating dendritic cells. Dendritic cells are also important in the rejection of foreign grafts (see Fig. 37).

Ly   Lymphocytes are often found in close contact with dendritic cells; this is presumably where antigen presentation and T–B cell cooperation take place (see Figs 17, 18).

S   The totipotent bone marrow stem cell, giving rise to all the cells found in blood.

PL   Blood platelets, though primarily involved in clotting, are able to phagocytose antigen–antibody complexes.

RBC   Antigen–antibody complexes which have bound complement can become attached to red blood cells via the CR1 receptor (see Fig. 5) on the latter, which then transport the complexes to the liver for removal by macrophages. This is sometimes referred to as 'immune adherence'.

PMN   Polymorphonuclear leucocyte, the major phagocytic cell of the blood; not, however, conventionally considered as part of the MPS.

Mono   Monocyte, formed in the marrow and travelling via the blood to the tissues, where it matures into a macrophage. It is likely, though not proved, that the specialized antigen-presenting cells also develop from monocytes.

Mac   Macrophage, the resident and long-lived tissue phagocyte. Macrophages may be either free in the tissues, or 'fixed' in the walls of blood sinuses, where they monitor the blood for particles, effete red cells, etc. This activity is strongest in the liver where the macrophages are called Kupffer cells. Macrophages in the lung alveoli are similarly responsible for keeping these vital air sacs free of particles and microbes. Macrophages (and polymorphs) have the valuable ability to recognize not only foreign matter but also antibody and/or complement bound to it, which greatly enhances phagocytosis (see Fig. 8). Despite their important role in host defense, the over-activation of macrophages is increasingly recognized as playing an important part in a very wide variety of chronic inflammatory conditions, including such common diseases as rheumatoid arthritis, Alzheimer's disease and atherosclerosis.

Sinus   Tortuous channels in liver, spleen, etc., through which blood passes to reach the veins, allowing the lining macrophages to remove damaged or antibody-coated cells and other particles. This process is so effective that a large injection, for example, carbon particles, can be removed from the blood within minutes, leaving the liver and spleen visibly black.

Microglia   The phagocytic cells of the brain, thought to be derived from incoming blood monocytes.

Lysozyme   An important antibacterial enzyme secreted into the blood by macrophages. Macrophages also produce other 'natural' humoral factors such as interferon and many complement components, cytotoxic factors, etc.

Giant cell; **epithelioid cell**   Macrophage-derived cells typically found at sites of chronic inflammation; by coalescing into a solid mass, or **granuloma**, they localize and wall off irritant or indigestible materials (see Fig. 35). However, granulomas also play a major role in disease (e.g. in tuberculosis) by obstructing airways, and causing internal bleeding.

8 Phagocytosis

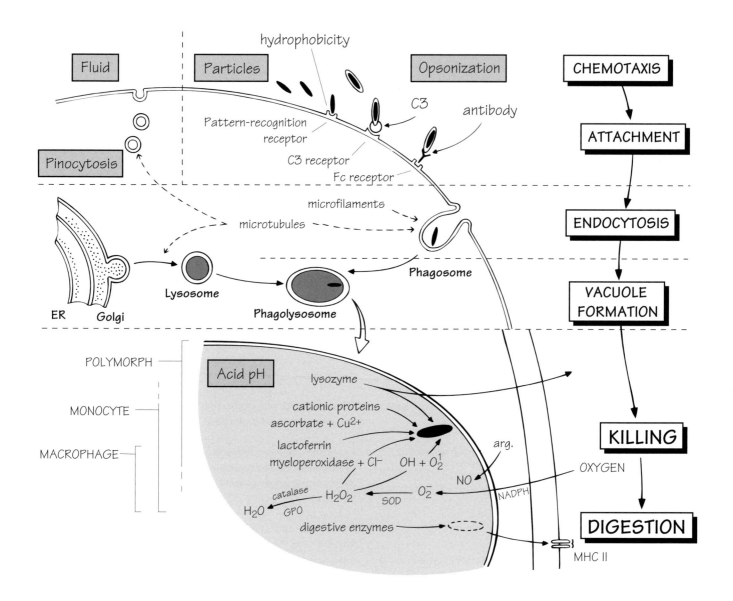

Numerous cells are able to ingest foreign materials, but the ability to increase this activity in response to opsonization by antibody and/or complement, so as to acquire antigen-specificity, is restricted to cells of the myeloid series, principally the **polymorphs**, **monocytes** and **macrophages**; these are sometimes termed 'professional' phagocytes.

Apart from some variations in their content of lysosomal enzymes, all myeloid cells use essentially similar mechanisms to phagocytose foreign objects, consisting of a sequence of **attachment** (top), endocytosis or **ingestion** (centre), and **digestion** (bottom). In the figure this process is shown for a typical bacterium (small black rods). In general, bacteria with **capsules** (shown outlined) are not phagocytosed unless opsonized, whereas many non-capsulated ones do not require this. There are certain differences between phagocytic cells; for example polymorphs are very short-lived (hours or days) and often die in the process of phagocytosis, while macrophages, which lack some of the more destructive enzymes, usually survive to phagocytose again. Also, macrophages can actively secrete some of their enzymes, e.g. lysozyme. There are surprisingly large species differences in the proportions of the various lysosomal enzymes.

Several of the steps in phagocytosis shown in the figure may be specifically defective for genetic reasons (see Fig. 39), as well as being actively inhibited by particular micro-organisms (see Figs 27–29). In either case the result is a failure to eliminate micro-organisms or foreign material properly, leading to chronic infection and/or chronic inflammation.

Chemotaxis The process by which cells are attracted towards bacteria, etc., often by following a gradient of molecules released by the microbe (see Fig. 6).

Pinocytosis 'Cell drinking'; the ingestion of soluble materials, conventionally applied to particles under 1 μm in diameter.

Hydrophobicity Hydrophobic groups tend to attach to the hydrophobic surface of cells; this may explain the 'recognition' of damaged cells, denatured proteins, etc. Bacterial capsules, largely polysaccharide, reduce hydrophobicity and block attachment, an important escape mechanism used by many of the most virulent bacteria (see Fig. 27).

Pattern-recognition receptors Phagocytic cells have surface structures which recognize complementary molecular structures on the surface of common pathogens. Examples are the mannose-receptors (mannose is a major component of the cell wall of many micro-organisms, but is rarely found exposed on the surface of vertebrate cells), and the lipopolysaccharide (LPS) receptors.

C3 receptor Phagocytic cells (and some lymphocytes) can bind C3b, produced from C3 by activation by bacteria, etc., either directly or via antibody (see Fig. 5 for details of the receptors).

Fc receptor Phagocytic cells (and most lymphocytes, platelets, etc.) can bind the Fc portion of antibody, especially of the IgG class.

Opsonization refers to the promotion or enhancement of attachment via the C3 or Fc receptor. Discovered by Almroth Wright and made famous by G.B. Shaw in *The Doctor's Dilemma*, opsonization is probably the single most important process by which antibody helps to overcome infections, particularly bacterial.

Phagosome A vacuole formed by the internalization of surface membrane along with an attached particle.

Microtubules Short rigid structures composed of the protein tubulin which arrange themselves into channels for vacuoles, etc. to travel within the cell, and also serve to stiffen the membrane.

Microfilaments Contractile protein (actin) filaments responsible for membrane activities such as pinocytosis and phagosome formation. There are also intermediate filaments composed of the protein vimentin.

ER Endoplasmic reticulum; a membranous system of sacs and tubules with which ribosomes are associated in the synthesis of many proteins for secretion.

Golgi The region where products of the ER are packaged into vesicles (see also Fig. 17).

Lysosome A membrane-bound package of hydrolytic enzymes usually active at acid pH (e.g. acid phosphatase, DNAase). Lysosomes are found in almost all cells, and are vehicles for secretion as well as digestion. They are prominent in macrophages and polymorphs, which also have separate vesicles containing lysozyme and other enzymes; together with lysosomes these constitute the **granules** whose staining patterns characterize the various types of polymorph (neutrophil, basophil, eosinophil). Newly formed lysosomes not containing any substrate are sometimes called 'primary'.

Phagolysosome A vacuole formed by the fusion of a phagosome and lysosome(s), in which micro-organisms are killed and digested.

Lactoferrin A protein that inhibits bacteria by depriving them of iron, which it binds with an extremely high affinity.

Cationic proteins Examples are 'phagocytin', 'leukin'; microbicidal agents found in some polymorph granules. Eosinophils are particularly rich in cationic proteins, which can be secreted when the cell 'degranulates', making them highly cytotoxic cells.

Ascorbate interacts with copper ions and hydrogen peroxide, and can be bactericidal.

Oxygen Intracellular killing of many bacteria requires the uptake of oxygen by the phagocytic cell, i.e. it is 'aerobic'. Through a series of enzyme reactions including NADPH oxidase and superoxide dismutase (SOD) this oxygen is progressively reduced to superoxide (O^-_2), hydrogen peroxide (H_2O_2) and hydroxyl ions (**OH**) and singlet oxygen (O^1_2). These 'free radicals' are highly toxic to many micro-organisms but they act only briefly because of cellular enzymes such as **catalase** and glutathione peroxidase (**GPO**) which remove them. Not surprisingly, some bacteria make such enzymes too (see Fig. 27). Nitric oxide (**NO**) produced from arginine is another reactive oxygen-containing compound which is highly toxic to micro-organisms when produced in large amounts by activated macrophages. In contrast much lower levels of nitric oxide are produced constitutively by endothelial cells, and play a key role in the regulation of blood-vessel tone.

Myeloperoxidase An important microbicidal enzyme in conjunction with hydrogen peroxide and halide (e.g. chloride) ions. It is absent from mature macrophages but may be partly replaced by catalase.

Lysozyme (muramidase) lyses many saprophytes (e.g. *Micrococcus lysodeicticus*) and some pathogenic bacteria damaged by antibody and/or complement. It is a major secretory product of macrophages, present in the blood at levels of micrograms per ml.

Digestive enzymes The enzymes by which lysosomes are usually identified, such as acid phosphatase, lipase, elastase, β glucuronidase, and the cathepsins thought to be important in antigen processing via the **MHC** Class II pathway (see Fig. 17).

9 Lymphocytes

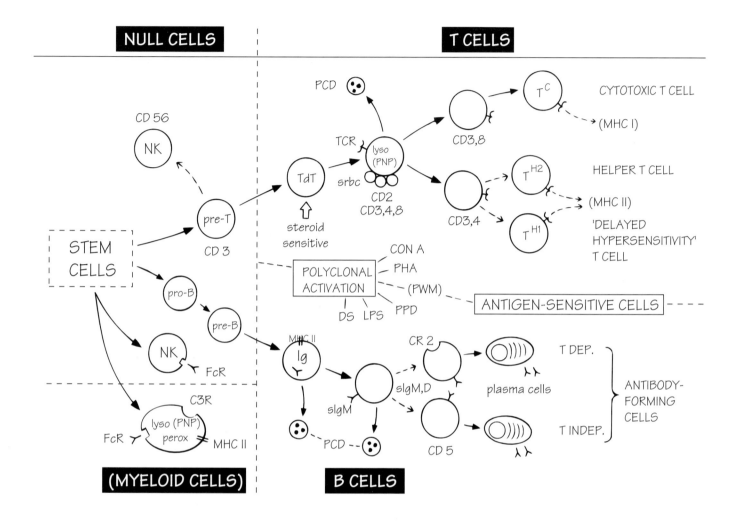

NULL CELLS

T CELLS

CD 56

NK

STEM CELLS

pre-T

CD 3

pro-B

pre-B

NK

FcR

C3R

FcR

lyso (PNP) perox

MHC II

(MYELOID CELLS)

PCD

TCR

TdT

srbc

steroid sensitive

CD2
CD3,4,8

lyso (PNP)

CD3,8

CD3,4

T^C

T^{H2}

T^{H1}

CYTOTOXIC T CELL

(MHC I)

HELPER T CELL

(MHC II)

'DELAYED HYPERSENSITIVITY' T CELL

CON A
PHA
(PWM)
PPD

POLYCLONAL ACTIVATION

DS   LPS

ANTIGEN-SENSITIVE CELLS

MHC II

Ig

sIgM

PCD

CR 2

sIgM,D

plasma cells

CD 5

T DEP.

T INDEP.

ANTIBODY-FORMING CELLS

B CELLS

As befits the cell of adaptive immunity, the lymphocyte has several unique features: restricted receptors permitting each cell to respond to an individual antigen (the basis of **specificity**), clonal proliferation and long life span (the basis of **memory**), and recirculation from the tissues back into the bloodstream, which ensures that specific memory following a local response has a bodywide **distribution**.

The discovery in the early 1960s of the two major lymphocyte subpopulations, **T** (thymus-dependent; top) and **B** (bursa or bone marrow-dependent; bottom), had roughly the same impact on cellular immunology as the double helix on molecular biology. The first property of T cells to be distinguished was that of 'helping' B cells to make antibody, but further subdivisions have subsequently come to light, based on both functional and physical differences; three, and possibly four types of T cell are now recognized (top right). In the figure, the main surface features (or 'markers') of the various stages of lymphocyte differentiation are given, using mainly the CD classification (see Section 44) but also indicating where some other important surface molecules first make their appearance.

Cells resembling lymphocytes, but without characteristic T or B cell

markers are referred to as 'null' (left). This group probably includes early T cells, B cells and monocytes, as well as the 'natural killer' cells possibly important in tumour and virus immunity. In blood and lymphoid organs, up to 10% of lymphocytes are 'null'.

One of the most exciting developments in biology was the discovery that it is possible to perpetuate individual lymphocytes by fusing them with a tumour cell. In the case of B lymphocytes, this can mean an endless supply of individual, or **monoclonal**, antibodies, which has had far-reaching applications in the diagnosis and treatment of disease and the study of cell surfaces. Indeed, the classification of lymphocytes themselves, and of most other cells too, is now mainly based on patterns of reactivity with a large range of monoclonal typing antibodies (see Appendix 3, Section 44).

In the case of T cells, it is also possible to keep them proliferating indefinitely in culture by judicious application of their specific antigen and non-specific growth factors such as IL-2 (see Fig. 23). The properties of the resulting **lines** or **clones** have given much information on the regulation of normal T cell function.

Natural killer cells

NK Natural killer cells are cytotoxic to some virus-infected cells and some tumours (see also Fig. 26). NK cells express a special class of polymorphic receptors which bind self-MHC and then negatively signal to the cell to prevent activation of cytotoxicity. NK cells are therefore only activated when cells lose expression of MHC molecules, such as sometimes occurs during viral infection or tumour growth. They thus form an important counterpart to **cytotoxic T cells** (see below) which kill cells only when they *do* express MHC molecules. NK cells are generally believed to represent a lymphocyte lineage, like B and T cells. Monocytes, macrophages and granulocytes can also be effective in cytotoxicity, but this is dependent on an antibody–mediated interaction (ADCC). Collectively, these are sometimes referred to as **K** cells. **K** cells carry the 'Fc receptor'; a receptor for the Fc portion of antibody, especially IgG, which links the ADCC effector cell to its target.

T cells

TdT Terminal deoxynucleotidyl transferase, a DNA polymerase found mainly in cortical, and therefore young, thymocytes, involved in generating diversity in the genes for the T cell receptor.

TCR The T cell receptor for antigen, analogous to surface Ig on the B cell (see Fig. 14). Two alternative types of T cell receptor exist, consisting either of a dimer made up of an α and a β chain or, in a small proportion of T cells a $\gamma\delta$ dimer.

PNP Purine nucleoside phosphorylase, a purine salvage enzyme, found in human T cells and monocytes, but not B cells; a potentially useful marker (see also Fig. 39).

Lyso Lysosomal enzymes (e.g. acid phosphatase, esterases, etc.) are found in myeloid cells and to a lesser extent in T cells.

CD Based on reactivity with various monoclonal antibodies recognizing surface molecules. T and B cells can be classified and their lineages worked out. A full list of CD numbers is given in Appendix 3 (Section 44), but it should be noted that some of the older functional names (C3 receptor, sheep-cell receptor, etc.) are still in use.

Polyclonal activation Stimulation of a substantial number of lymphocytes, i.e. many clones, rather than the few or single clones normally stimulated by an antigen. Since the first sign of activation is often mitosis, polyclonal activators are sometimes known as 'mitogens'. A surprising number of such 'lectins' are of plant origin, e.g. concanavalin A (CON A) and phytohaemagglutinin (PHA), and act by a complementary interaction with surface carbohydrates on the cell, whose real function is probably to recognize microbial structures.

SRBC Sheep red blood cell. Most human T cells bind sheep RBC via the CD2 molecule, to make 'rosettes' *in vitro*. The T cells of many species react in the same way with selected heterologous erythrocytes (e.g. cat: guinea-pig). Like the response to mitogens, this is a useful marker without functional significance—which needs to be distinguished from the use of sheep red cells as *antigens*, very common in experimental immunology.

Cytotoxic T cell A key cell in virus immunity (see Figs 20, 26).

Helper T cell The CD4 T cell is essential for most antibody and cell-mediated responses (see Figs 17, 18, 20). CD4 T cells can be further subdivided on the basis of which cytokines they secrete. TH1 cells, for example, make cytokines such as γ-interferon important for driving cell-mediated immunity (CMI), or **delayed hypersensitivity.** In contrast, TH2 cells make cytokines needed for helping B cells to make antibody (such as IL-4).

B cells

Ig; sIg Immunoglobulin, at first cytoplasmic and later surface bound, is the key feature of B cells, through which they recognize specific antigens (see Figs 12, 15).

MHC II Antigens coded by the Class II region of the major histocompatibility complex, expressed mainly on B cells, macrophages and dendritic cells, and involved in the interaction of these with the CD4 type of T cells (see Figs 13, 14, 17).

CR2 Receptors for C3 on B cells may be involved in the generation of memory responses.

DS Dextran sulphate. **LPS** lipopolysaccharide, e.g. *Salmonella* endotoxin. **SA** *Staphylococcus aureus* cell wall. The above are normally mitogenic only for B cells, possibly at different stages.

PWM Pokeweed mitogen, mitogenic for both T and B cells when both are present. There is unfortunately no ideal mitogen for human B cells.

T dep., T indep. Some antibody formation, especially IgM, does not require T cell help, and is called 'thymus independent'. It usually involves direct cross-linking of antibody on the B cell surface by multivalent antigens like bacterial cell wall polysaccharides.

PCD Programmed cell death, also known as *apoptosis*; a process by which cells are induced to die without damage to surrounding tissue. A very high proportion of both B and T cells die in this way because they fail to rearrange their receptor genes properly, or because they threaten to be 'self-reactive' (see Fig. 36).

10 Primary lymphoid organs and lymphopoiesis

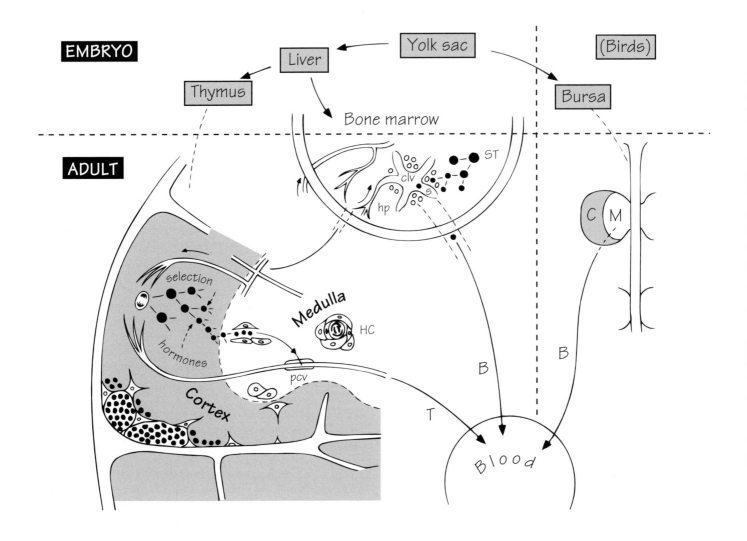

The first strong evidence for distinct lymphocyte populations was the complementary effects in birds of early removal of the **thymus** (which mainly affects cell-mediated immunity) and the **bursa of Fabricius** (which affects antibody responses). A continuing puzzle has been the identification of what represents the bursa in mammals; despite a phase when 'gut-associated lymphoid tissue' was a popular candidate, current opinion considers there to be no true analogue, the liver taking over the function of B cell maturation in the fetus, the bone marrow in the adult.

The production of both B and T lymphocytes is a highly random and, at first glance, wasteful process, quite unlike any other form of haemopoiesis. It involves the rearrangement of genes to give each cell a unique receptor molecule (see Figs 14 and 15 for details) and the elimination of all those cells which fail to achieve this, plus those that carry re-

ceptors which would recognize 'self' molecules and thus be potentially self-destructive (see Fig. 36). Since recognition by T cells is more complex, involving the MHC as well as foreign antigen (see Figs 13, 14, 17), production of T cells is a correspondingly more elaborate process, requiring two separate selection steps, one *for* self MHC and one *against* self antigens.

There are still some controversies surrounding the thymus. Do the thymus 'hormones' function only in the organ, or do they have a true endocrine role elsewhere? Are the Hassal's corpuscles the site of cell destruction? How is the same receptor selected twice, in opposite directions? Is the thymus something to do with ageing? (One wonders how long it will be before someone revives Galen's theory that it is the site of the soul!)

Yolk sac

The source of the earliest haemopoietic tissue, including the lymphocyte precursors.

Bursa

In birds, B lymphocytes differentiate in the bursa of Fabricius, a cloacal outgrowth with many crypts and follicles, which reaches its maximum size a few weeks after birth and thereafter atrophies. Despite claims for the appendix, tonsil, etc., there is probably no mammalian analogue.

M Medulla; the region where the first stem cells colonize the bursal follicles.

C Cortex; the site of proliferation of the B lymphocytes.

Liver

During fetal life in mammals, the major haemopoietic and lymphopoietic organ.

Bone marrow

ST Stem cells for the B cell series.

HP Haemopoietic area. The anatomical location of lymphopoiesis in liver and bone marrow is not exactly known, but it presumably proceeds alongside the other haemopoietic pathways, in close association with macrophages and stromal cells. At least 70% of B cells die before release, probably because of faulty rearrangement of their immunoglobulin genes (see Figs 9, 15) or excessive self-reactivity.

S Sinus, collecting differentiated cells for discharge into the blood via the central longitudinal vein (**CLV**).

Thymus

A two-lobed organ lying in the upper chest (in birds, in the neck), derived from outgrowths of the third and fourth branchial cleft and pharyngeal pouch. Like the bursa, it is largest in early life, though its subsequent atrophy is slower. In it, bone marrow-derived stem cells are converted into mature T lymphocytes.

Hormones Numerous soluble factors extracted from the thymus have been shown to stimulate the maturation of T cells, as judged by function or surface markers or both. There is no agreed terminology, and the following list is far from complete:
- Thymosin α1 (MW 3108), β1 (MW 8451), β4 (MW 4982)
- Thymopoietin I, II (MW 9562)
- Thymosin (MW 3108), B (MW 8451), B4 (MW 4982)
- Thymic humoral factor (MW 3220)
- Thymostimulin (MW 12 000)
- Facteur thymique serique (MW 857).

Cortex Dark-staining outer part packed with lymphocytes, compartmentalized by elongated epithelial cells. The process of proliferation and selection occurs mainly here.

Medulla Inner, predominantly epithelial part, to which cortical lymphocytes migrate before export via venules and lymphatics. The final stages of selection may occur at the cortico-medullary junction.

PCV Post-capillary venule, through which lymphocytes enter the thymic veins and ultimately the blood.

HC Hassal's corpuscle—a structure peculiar to the thymus, in which epithelial cells become concentrically compressed and keratinized, possibly the site of removal of apoptotic cells.

Selection Because of its importance and complexity, the process of selecting T lymphocytes for export has attracted intense study, and is currently considered to consist of the following stages: (i) CD4– CD8– ('double negative') cells proliferate in the outer region of the cortex, during which they become CD4+ CD8+ (double positive) and rearrange their TCR genes; (ii) under the influence of thymic stromal cells, T lymphocytes whose TCR recognizes one of the available 'self' MHC molecules (see Figs 13, 14) survive, and the rest die; (iii) cells that recognize an MHC Class I molecule lose CD4 and retain CD8; those that recognize an MHC Class II molecule lose CD8 and retain CD4; thus they are now 'single positives'; (iv) under the influence of dendritic cells presenting 'self' antigens, in the form of short peptides (see Fig. 17 for details), potentially self-reactive T cells are eliminated; (v) the remainder, probably only about 2% of the starting population, are allowed to exit, and these make up the peripheral T lymphocyte pool.

11 Secondary lymphoid organs and lymphocyte traffic

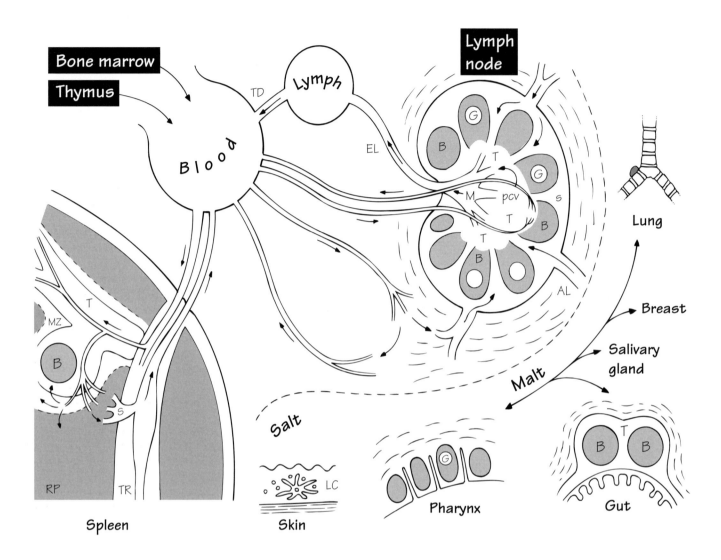

The ability to **recirculate** from blood to tissues and back through the lymphoid system is unique to lymphocytes and, coupled with their long life span and specificity for individual antigens, equips them for their central role in adaptive immune responses.

The thorough mixing of lymphocytes, particularly in the **spleen** and **lymph nodes**, ensures the maximum contact of antigen-presenting cells that have newly encountered antigen, with T and B lymphocytes potentially able to respond, which would otherwise be a very rare event. The bodywide dissemination of expanded T and B populations in readiness for a second encounter with the same antigen ensures that 'memory' is available at all sites.

There is a tendency for different types of lymphocyte to 'home' to different regions in the lymphoid organs (**T** and **B** areas in the figure; B areas are shaded). This is presumably due to either chemotactic factors unique

to particular sites, or to recognition of different lymphocytes by local elements such as adhesion molecules on the inner surface of the vascular endothelium or the dendritic antigen-presenting cells (not shown here, but see Fig. 7).

In general, lymph nodes respond to antigens introduced into the tissues they drain, and the spleen responds to antigens in the blood. The gut, lungs, breast, and external mucous surfaces also have their own less specialized lymphoid areas which to some extent behave as a separate circuit for recirculation purposes and are often known as the **mucosa-associated lymphoid tissues** or MALT. These can be further subdivided into gut-(GALT), bronchial (BALT) and skin-associated (SALT) lymphoid tissue. In each case, the objective seems to be to provide a local lymphoid system specialized for the antigens most likely to be encountered there.

Lymph node

Lymph nodes (or 'glands') constitute the main bulk of the organized lymphoid tissue. They are strategically placed so that lymph from most parts of the body drains through a series of nodes before reaching the thoracic duct (**TD**), which empties into the left subclavian vein to allow the lymphocytes to recirculate again via the blood.

AL, EL   Afferent and efferent lymphatics, through which lymph passes from the tissues to peripheral and then central lymph nodes.

S   Lymphatic sinus, through which lymph flows from the afferent lymphatic into the cortical and medullary sinuses.

M   Medullary sinus, collecting lymph for exit via the efferent lymphatic. It is in the medulla that antibody formation takes place and plasma cells are prominent.

G   Germinal centre; an area of larger cells that develops within the follicle after antigenic stimulation. It is thought to be the site of B memory-cell generation, and contains special follicular dendritic cells which retain antigens on their surface for weeks and perhaps even years (see Fig. 18 for further details).

T   T cell area, or 'paracortex', largely occupied by T cells but through which B cells travel to reach the medulla. The dendritic cells here are specialized for presentation of antigen to T cells, and are probably the site where T and B lymphocytes of the right specificity meet and co-operate — which would otherwise be a very rare event.

PCV   Post-capillary venule; a specialized small venule with high cuboidal endothelium through which lymphocytes leave the blood to enter the paracortex and thence the efferent lymphatic.

Spleen

The spleen differs from a lymph node in having no lymphatic drainage, and also in containing large numbers of red cells. In some species it can act as an erythropoietic organ or a reservoir for blood.

TR   Trabecula(e); connective tissue structures sheathing the vessels, especially veins.

T   T cell area; the lymphoid sheath surrounding the arteries is mostly composed of T lymphocytes.

B   B cell area, or lymphoid follicle, typically lying to one side of the lymphoid sheath. Germinal centres are commonly found in the follicle, alongside the follicular artery.

MZ   Marginal zone, the region between the lymphoid areas and the red pulp, where lymphocytes chiefly leave the blood to enter the lymphoid areas, and red cells and plasma cells to enter the red pulp.

RP   Red pulp; a reticular meshwork through which blood passes to enter the venous sinusoids, and in which surveillance and removal of damaged red cells is thought to occur. For contrast, the lymphoid areas are sometimes called 'white pulp'. Macrophages in the red pulp and in the marginal zone can retain antigens, as the dendritic cells in the lymph nodes do. As in the medulla of the lymph node, plasma cells are frequent.

S   Sinusoids, the large sacs which collect blood for return via the splenic vein.

Mucosa-associated lymphoid tissues

At least 50% of all tissue lymphocytes are associated with mucosal surfaces, emphasizing that these are the main sites of entry of foreign material. It is estimated that the total area of mucosal surfaces is 400 times that of the body.

Gut   The GALT is composed of two types of tissue: *organized* and *diffuse*. Typical organized tissues are the lymphoid aggregates, e.g. the Peyer's patches, where antigens are first encountered, analogous to the lymphoid follicles in lymph nodes. The actual transfer of antigens from the gut lumen to the subepithelial area occurs via specialized M (membrane) cells, which pass them to dendritic cells where they are presented to T and B cells in the normal way. Most of the B cells are specialized for IgA production, and B-cell memory develops in germinal centres. Cells that leave the follicles circulate in the blood to the diffuse lymphoid areas in the **lamina propria,** where large numbers of IgA plasma cells are found, as well as CD8 +, γδ T cells, NK cells, and mast cells. This preferential homing of MALT cells to MALT sites is mediated by specialized surface molecules on the lymphocytes and on the endothelium of blood vessel walls.

IgA   Lamina propria B cells are responsible for the majority of gA antibody, although a small amount is made in other sites such as bone marrow. IgA occurs mainly as dimers of two molecules held together by a J (joining) chain (see Fig. 16). IgA is protected against proteolytic digestion by a polypeptide **secretory piece** derived from the poly Ig receptor and added to the IgA dimers in the epithelial cells.

Pharynx   Lymphoid aggregates are prominent at this vulnerable site (tonsil and adenoids). The salivary glands also contain lymphocytes of MALT origin.

Lung   The lung alveoli are largely protected from inhaled antigens by the upward movement of mucus propelled by beating cilia and ultimately coughed up or swallowed (the 'muco-ciliary escalator'). However, organized and diffuse lymphoid tissues are also present in the walls of the bronchi.

Skin   Antigens entering via the skin can reach the local lymph node by being taken up in Langerhans cells (**LC** in figure, and see Fig. 7), which can pass from the skin to the node, where they probably settle in the T cell areas. LC are extremely sensitive to UV light, which may be why UV reduces contact sensitivity reactions and conceivably also why it facilitates the induction of suppressor rather than helper T cells (see Fig. 31 for the significance of this in relation to skin cancer).

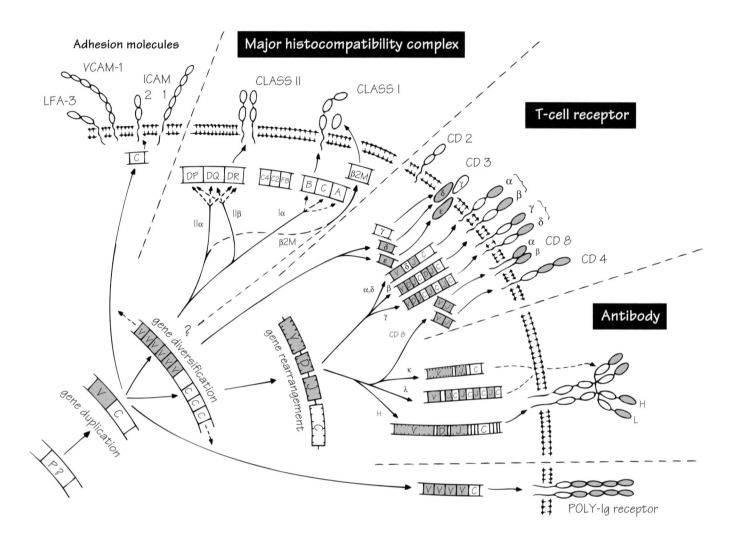

At this point it may be worth re-emphasizing the difference between 'natural' and 'adaptive' immunity, which lies essentially in the degree of **discrimination** of the respective recognition systems.

Natural immune recognition, e.g. by phagocytic cells, NK cells, or the alternative complement pathway, while incompletely understood and extremely interesting, appears to be based on relatively simple distinctions: generally speaking, a particular foreign material is either recognized and dealt with or not: a 'friend or foe' approach.

Recognition by **lymphocytes**, the fundamental cells of adaptive immunity, is quite another matter. An enormous range of foreign substances can be individually distinguished and the appropriate response set in motion. This is only possible because of the evolution of three sets of **cell-surface receptors**, each showing extensive heterogeneity, namely the **antibody** molecule, the **T cell receptor** and the molecules of the **major histocompatibility complex** (MHC). Thanks to molecular biology, the fascinating discovery has been made that all these receptors share enough sequences, at both the gene (DNA) and protein (amino acid) level, to make it clear that they have evolved from a single precursor, presumably a primitive recognition molecule of some kind (see Fig. 3).

Because antibody was the first of these genetic systems to be identified, they are often collectively referred to as the **immunoglobulin gene superfamily**, which contains other related molecules too, some with immunological functions, some at present without. What they all share is a structure based on a number of folded sequences about 110 amino acids long and featuring β-pleated sheets, called **domains** (shown in the figure as oval loops protruding from the cell membrane).

Much work is still needed to fill in the evolutionary gaps, and the figure can only give an impression of what the relationships between this remarkable family of molecules may have been. Their present-day structure and function are considered in more detail in the following four figures.

P?   The precursor gene from which the Ig superfamily is presumed to have evolved. It has not been identified in any existing species, but possibly it coded for a self-recognizing molecule such as that used by sponges (see Fig. 3). However, invertebrates appear to use a variety of other recognition molecules to trigger responses to pathogens. These include lectins, which recognize patterns of sugars commonly expressed on the surface of invading micro-organisms (see Fig. 8).

V, C   A vital early step seems to have been the duplication of this gene into two, one of which became the parent of all present-day **variable** (V) genes and the other of **constant** (C) genes. In the figure, the genes and polypeptides with significant enough homology to be considered part of the V gene family are shown shaded. Subsequent further duplications, with diversification among different V and C genes, led ultimately to the large variety of present-day domains.

Major histocompatibility complex   The genes shown are those found in man, also known as HLA (human leucocyte antigen) genes. They code for two types of cell-surface molecule found on all nucleated cells (Class I) or some immunological cells only (Class II). Their α and β chains contain constant regions but it is not certain whether the outer domains are derived from V genes. Interactions between MHC molecules and T cell receptors are vital to all adaptive immune responses. There are quite large species differences in the numbers of MHC gene loci, but it has been calculated that the six of humans are close to optimal. Interestingly, during metamorphosis of amphibians, Class II antigens appear before Class I.

β2M   β2 microglobulin, which combines with Class I chains to complete the four-domain molecule. The ancestry of this molecule is still in doubt.

C2, C4, FB   Three complement components which, rather surprisingly, are coded for by genes lying within the MHC, but are structurally quite unrelated to MHC molecules.

Gene rearrangement   A process found only in T and B cells, through which an enormous degree of receptor diversity is generated by bringing together one V gene, one J gene (and one D gene in the case of IgH chains), each from a set containing from two to over a hundred. It involves excisions of DNA and results in a messenger RNA in which further excisions lead to a polypeptide chain composed of only one combination out of the possible thousands. Since a unique gene rearrangement occurs in each T and B cell, and is then inherited in the progeny, each lymphocyte or clone of lymphocytes is effectively unique—which forms the basis for all adaptive immune responses (see Figs 17–20).

T cell receptor (TCR)   A complex of T cell surface molecules, including TCR α plus β, or γ plus δ chains, CD3 and CD4 or CD8, depending on the type of T cell. Together these form a unit which enables the T cell to recognize a specific antigen plus a particular MHC molecule, to become activated and to carry out its function (help, cytotoxicity, etc.).

Antibody   The antibody or immunoglobulin molecule plays the part of cell-surface receptor on B lymphocytes as well as being secreted in vast amounts by activated B cells to give rise to serum antibody—a vital part of defence against infectious organisms. The domains are fairly similar to those of the T cell receptor α and β chains, but assembled in a different way, with 2 four-domain heavy (H) chains bonded to 2 two-domain light (L) chains.

Note that the process of diversification in the genes for the various chains has not always proceeded in the same way. For example, mammalian heavy and light (κ) chains have all their J genes together, between V and C, while light (λ) chains have repeated J–C segments and sharks have the whole V–D–J–C segment duplicated—a considerably less efficient arrangement for generating the maximum diversity.

Poly Ig receptor   A molecule found on some epithelial cells which helps to transport antibody into secretions such as mucus. Many other molecules show traces of the characteristic domain structure, including some Fc receptors, adhesion molecules (see below) and receptors for growth factors and cytokines. The common feature seems to be an involvement in cell–cell interactions, with the 'breakaway' immunoglobulin molecule the exception rather than the rule.

Killer Inhibitory Receptors (KIR)   Immunoglobulin-family receptors are found on Natural Killer cells (see Fig. 9). They recognize MHC molecules on target cells and send negative signals to the NK cells which inhibit their activation, and hence prevent killing of targets. NK cells are therefore active only against cells which have lost MHC expression, either as a result of infection (e.g. by viruses) or as a result of malignant transformation (i.e. cancer cells). Some NK cells also express other negative receptors which belong to a different structural family of molecules known as C-lectins. But a common feature of all NK negative receptors is the presence of an inhibitory signalling motif (known as an Immunoreceptor Tyrosine-based Inhibitory Motif, ITIM) on their cytoplasmic tails which plays an important role in the signal-transduction process.

Adhesion molecules   Already mentioned in connection with inflammation (see Fig. 6), a large range of surface molecules help to hold cells together and facilitate cell–cell interactions or binding to blood vessel walls. Some of these, as shown in the figure, belong to the immunoglobulin superfamily, and they usually bind to one or a small number of corresponding 'ligands'. Some examples of pairs of molecules important in adhesion are shown below, with those belonging to the immunoglobulin superfamily shown in bold. Many of these molecules have both 'common' names and CD numbers (see p. 94).

Adhesion molecules	Ligand	Function of interaction
CD2	**CD58 (LFA3)**	T cell/antigen presenting cell
VCAM-1	VLA-4	Leukocyte/endothelium and Leukocyte/Leukocyte
ICAM-1 (CD54) **ICAM-2 (CD102)** **ICAM-3 (CD50)**	LFA-1	Leukocyte/endothelium and T cell/antigen presenting cell
P-selectin L-selectin E-selectin	Vascular addressins, mucin-like molecules (CD34, MadCAM-1, GlyCAM-1)	Leukocyte/endothelium

VCAM, vascular cell adhesion molecule; ICAM, intercellular adhesion molecule.

13 The major histocompatibility complex

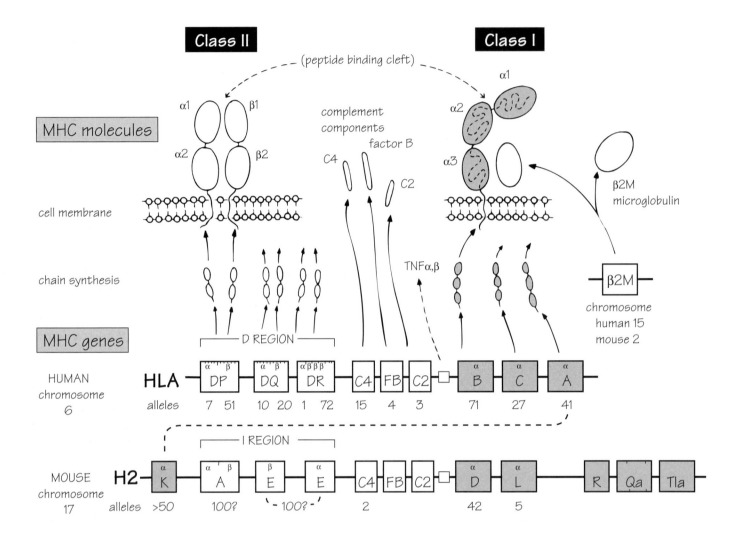

This large and important set of genes owes its rather clumsy-sounding name to the fact that the proteins it codes for were first detected by their effect on transplant rejection—that is, tissue *incompatibility*. However, it is now clear that their real purpose is to act as 'identity markers' on the surface of the various cells with which T lymphocytes need to interact, via their own receptors, in carrying out their adaptive immunological functions.

Again for historical reasons, the MHC in the mouse (extreme bottom line in the figure) is known as **H-2**, while in man it is called **HLA** ('human leucocyte antigen'). In fact the basic layout of the MHC genes is remarkably similar in all animals so far studied, consisting of a set of Class I (shaded in the figure) and a set of Class II genes, differing slightly in structure and in the way they interact with T cells (see Fig. 14).

In the figure the names of genes are shown boxed, while the numbers below indicate the number of alternative versions or **alleles** which can occur at each locus. Clearly there is enormous polymorphism throughout the whole MHC, and the number of possible combinations on a single chromosome probably exceeds 3×10^6, so that an individual, with a set of MHC molecules coded for by both chromosomes, can have any one of about 10^{13} combinations, which is part of the problem in transplanting kidneys, etc. (see Fig. 37).

Since HLA typing became a routine procedure, it has emerged that many diseases are significantly commoner, or sometimes rarer, in people of a particular HLA type. There are several mechanisms which might account for this but none of them has yet been established to everybody's satisfaction.

H2 The MHC of the mouse, carried on chromosome 17. There are at least 20 other minor histocompatibility genes on other chromosomes, numbered H1, H3, H4, etc. but H2 is by far the strongest in causing transplant rejection and the only one known to be involved in normal cell interactions.

K, D, L The Class I genes of H2, coding for the α chain (MW 44 000), which in combination with β2 microglobulin (see below) makes up the four-domain K, D and L molecules or 'antigens'. The N-terminal portions of the α chains are extremely variable, having probably evolved to interact with different viruses. Because any cell can potentially be infected by a virus, Class I antigens are expressed on virtually all cells in the body, with the exception of red blood cells in some species. The number of different alleles known is shown below each locus, but these are no doubt underestimates.

A, E The classical Class II genes of H2, which present processed peptide antigen to the antigen receptor of CD4 T cells (Figs 17, 18 & 20). A and E contain separate genes for the α (MW 33 000) and β (MW 28 000) chains of the four-domain molecule. Unlike Class I, Class II molecules are expressed only on a minority of cells, namely those which T cells need to interact with and regulate (see Fig. 14).

HLA The human MHC, on chromosome 6, closely analogous to H2 except that the Class I genes lie together and there are three Class II genes.

A, B, C The classical human Class I genes which present processed peptide antigens to the antigen receptor of CD8 T cells. A is the homologue of K in the mouse.

DP, DQ, DR The classical human Class II genes which present processed peptide antigens to the antigen receptor of CD4 T cells. The distribution of these different isoforms within the body is slightly different, but it is still unclear whether each one plays a distinct role in the regulation of T cell responses.

Peptide binding cleft The classical MHC I and II molecules contain a peptide binding site at the distal end of the molecule from the membrane. This peptide binding site is formed by two protein α-helices, lying on top of a β-pleated sheet. The binding site, or groove as it is often known, can accommodate a peptide of about 9–10 amino acids in length, although for class II MHC molecules, the ends of the groove are open allowing longer peptides to extend out of either end. A wide variety of different peptides can be bound tightly, by interaction between conserved residues in the MHC molecules and the amino acid backbone of the antigen peptide. In order to accommodate the side-chains of the larger amino acids, however, the floor of the groove contains a number of pockets. It is the size and position of these pockets which limit the range of peptides which can be accommodated. This selectivity in peptide binding means that in each individual, only a small portion of each antigen can be presented to the T cells, focusing the immune response onto only a few defined epitopes.

Polymorphism The classical MHC genes in both human and mouse exist in many different allelic variants, making these genes the most polymorphic known. The differences between allelic forms are mostly within or close to the peptide-binding groove, and result in the different alleles binding to different peptide fragments from a particular protein antigen. Since MHC molecules are expressed codominantly (i.e. each cell expresses both paternally and maternally inherited alleles) this increases the number of antigens from each pathogen which can be presented to the immune system, and hence makes the immune response more vigorous. Some HLA alleles (for example A1 and B8) 'stay together' instead of segregating normally. This is called 'linkage disequilibrium' and may imply that such combinations are of survival value. Not all species show equally great MHC polymorphism—the Syrian hamster, for example, shows little class I variation, perhaps reflecting its isolated lifestyle and hence decreased susceptibility to viral epidemics.

Class IB genes Both human and mouse MHC loci encode a large number (around 50) of genes which code for proteins with a class I-like structure, known as class IB genes. These include Qa and Tla in the mouse, and E, F,G,H,J and X in the human. The function of many of these remains unknown, but some may play a part in controlling innate immunity, perhaps by regulating NK cell activation. Some class IB genes lie outside the MHC locus. One such family is the CD1 family, which plays a role in presenting mycobacterial cell-wall products.

The class II region As well as the classical class II genes involved in antigen presentation, the class II regions of both mouse and human genome contain genes encoding a number of other molecules involved in the antigen processing pathway (see Fig. 17). These include DM and DO (H2-O and H2-M in the mouse), class II MHC-like molecules which regulate the loading of peptide fragments onto DP, DQ and DR. The region also contains the LMP genes and the TAP genes (see Fig. 17).

C2, C4, FB These 'Class III' genes all code for complement components involved in the activation of C3. Curiously enough, these exist in several allelic forms, though this has no obvious significance. C4 can become attached to red cells and masquerade as a 'blood group'. Other genes located in this region include those coding for the adrenal enzyme 21-hydroxylase and for the cytokines TNFα and β.

β2M β2 microglobulin (MW 12 000) coded quite separately from the MHC, nevertheless forms part of all Class I molecules, stabilizing them on the cell surface. In the mouse there are two allelic forms, but in general β2M is one of the most remarkably conserved molecules known. It is also found free in the serum.

HLA-associated diseases Many diseases show genetic associations with particular HLA alleles. The most remarkable example is the rare sleep abnormality narcolepsy, which virtually only occurs in people carrying the DR2 antigen; the reason is quite unknown. After this, the most striking example is the group of arthropathies involving the sacroiliac joint (ankylosing spondylitis, Reiter's disease, etc.) where one HLA allele (B27) is found in up to 95% of cases—nearly 20 times its frequency in the general population. But numerous other diseases, including almost all of the autoimmune diseases, show a statistically significant association with particular HLA antigens or groups of antigens, especially in the class II region. The explanation probably lies in the ability or otherwise of the HLA molecule to present particular microbial peptides or, alternatively, self antigens. This whole field is still in an exciting stage of evolution.

14 The T cell receptor

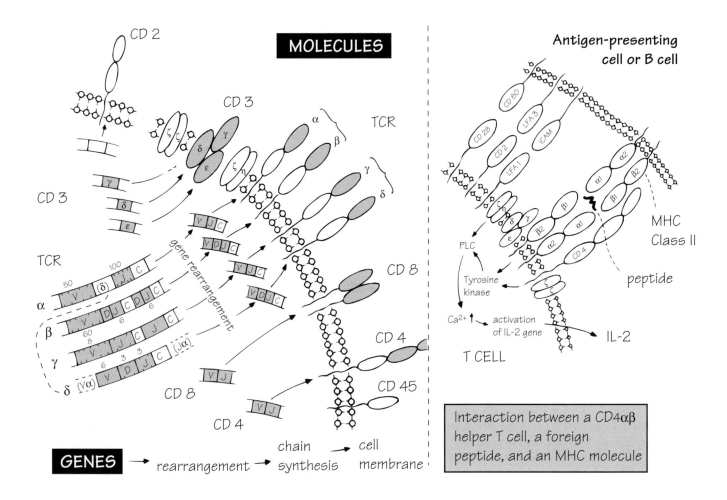

It has been evident for many years that T lymphocytes have a surface receptor for antigen, with roughly similar properties to the antibody on B lymphocytes, but furious controversy raged as to whether the two molecules were in fact identical. The issue was finally resolved in 1983–4 by the use of monoclonal antibodies to study the fine structure of the molecule and of DNA probing to identify the corresponding genes, and it is now clear that the T cell receptor (TCR) is a quite separate entity.

Like all members of the immunoglobulin superfamily, the T cell receptor has a structure of polypeptide chains made up of domains, linked together by disulphide bonds. In this case there are two major chains (α, β) each of two domains, but other molecules (e.g. CD4, CD8) also play a role in T cell interactions with MHC molecules, and a second (γδ) combination is found on some T cells instead of αβ. The way in which the TCR 'recognizes' a foreign antigen in association with an MHC molecule is illustrated in the right-hand part of the figure; in this case the T cell is of the helper variety. Knowledge of these interactions is far from complete, but advances are being made all the time: a particularly important breakthrough was the X-ray crystallography of a T cell receptor actually bound to an MHC/peptide complex. The α and β chains associate on the cell membrane with other trans-membrane proteins to form the CD3 complex. This complex is responsible for transducing an activation signal into the T cell.

An unusual feature of the α,β chains of the T cell receptor, which is shared with the heavy and light chain of the antibody molecule is that the genes for different parts of each polypeptide chain do not lie together on the chromosome, so that unwanted segments of DNA, and subsequently of RNA, have to be excised to bring them together. This process is known as **gene rearrangement** and occurs only in T and B cells, so that in all other cells the genes remain in their non-functional 'germ line' configuration. Once this rearrangement has occurred in an individual T lymphocyte, that cell is committed to a unique receptor, and therefore a unique antigen-recognizing ability. A similar thing happens to the immunoglobulin genes in B cells (see Fig. 15). In this and the following figure, the portions of genes and proteins which are shaded are those thought to have evolved from the primitive V region, though they do not all show the same degree of variability.

TCR The T cell receptor. It is made up of one α (MW 50 000) and one β (MW 45 000) chain, each with an outer variable domain, an inner constant domain and short intramembrane and cytoplasmic regions. Some T cells, especially early in fetal life and in some organs like the gut and skin, express the alternative γδ receptor and seem to recognize a different set of antigens from the αβ population. γδ T cells are rare in humans, but are a major proportion of T cells in other animals including cows, pigs and sheep. The way in which individual T cells are first positively and then negatively **selected** in the thymus to ensure they only recognize self MHC plus a foreign peptide is described in Fig. 10.

CD3 A complex of three chains, γ (MW 25 000), δ (MW 20 000), and ε (MW 20 000) which is essential to all T cell function. Also associated with the TCR–CD3 complex are two other signalling molecules, ζ and η. Interaction of antigen (i.e. MHC-plus-peptide) with this whole complex leads to **T cell activation** via a complex series of molecular steps still not completely understood.

CD4 A single-chain molecule (MW 60 000) found on human helper T cells. It interacts with MHC Class II molecules (as shown in the figure), and is therefore recruited into the vicinity of the T cell receptor, bringing with it a T-cell specific kinase, *lck*, which binds to its cytoplasmic portion, and which facilitates the process of T cell activation. CD4 is also the receptor which HIV uses to enter the T cell (see Fig. 40).

CD8 A 75 000 MW molecule found on most cytotoxic T cells. In man it is composed of two identical chains, but the equivalent in the mouse has two different chains (Ly2/3). It is involved in interacting with MHC Class I molecules. Because of their close association with the TCR, CD4 and CD8 are sometimes known as 'coreceptors'.

CD2, CD28 Binding of the T cell receptor to the MHC/peptide antigen is not, by itself, sufficient to activate T cells efficiently. T cells need simultaneously to receive signals via other cell-surface receptors, which bind ligands on the antigen presenting cell. Two examples of such **'co–stimulatory'** interactions are those between CD2 on the T cell, and LFA-3 (CD58) on the antigen presenting cell, and CD28 on the T cell and CD80 (B7.1) or CD86 (B7.2) on the antigen presenting cell. T cell activation therefore requires a simultaneous antigen specific interaction (between the TCR on the T cell and MHC/peptide on the antigen presenting cell) and a nonantigen specific co-stimulatory interaction. This is often called the 'two-signal' model of T cell activation (although in reality there are many more than two signals involved). It has important implications for the induction of tolerance (see Fig. 21) because when T cells recognize antigen in the absence of the right costimulation they can be unresponsive to future encounters with antigen (such T cells are described as **tolerant,** or sometimes **anergic).**

CD45 This transmembrane protein was originally known as 'leucocyte common antigen' because it is found on all white blood cells. However, on T cells, it has received much attention as a means of distinguishing 'memory' T cells (those which have already encountered antigen), from 'naïve' T cells (those which have yet to encounter antigens). The extra-cellular portion of CD45 exists in a number of variant forms. The shortest form (known as CD45Ro) is found on activated, and memory T cells, but not naïve T cells. In contrast, one of the longer forms (CD45RA) is found predominantly on naïve T cells. The ligand for the extracellular portion of CD45 is still unknown, but the intracellular portion codes for a tyrosine phosphatase, which plays a key part in TCR regulation via regulation of the tyrosine kinase *lck* (see above).

Gene rearrangement The TCR genes contain up to 100 V genes and numerous J genes, so that to make a single chain, one of each must be linked up to the correct C gene. This is done by excision of intervening DNA sequences and further excision in the messenger RNA, eventually producing a single V–D–J–C RNA to code for the polypeptide chain. When all the possible combinations of α and β chains are taken into account, the number of different TCR molecules available to an individual may be as high as 10^{10}. Note that the CD4 and CD8 genes, though apparently of V gene origin, do not rearrange and the molecules therefore do not show such diversity.

Antigen Shown in the figure as a short peptide, in this case bound by an MHC molecule and then recognized by the T cell receptor (for details see Fig. 17). If this recognition is strong enough, aided by CD4–MHC interaction, and the binding of costimulatory molecules on the T cell, T cell activation results. In the case of a cytotoxic T cell, a CD8 molecule would play the part of CD4, by interacting with MHC Class I molecules on the cell to be killed. Interestingly, some antigen peptides (antagonist peptides) can have the opposite effect, in that they somehow turn off T cell activation and make the T cells unresponsive to further stimulation. Such peptides might have possible therapeutic uses in regulating unwanted immune reactions such as allergies or autoimmunity.

T cell activation T cell activation is a complex series of molecular steps which follow the binding of the TCR to antigen, and which ultimately result in the transcription of some two hundred genes which determine T cell proliferation, differentiation and effector function. A key early event is the movement of many T cell receptor molecules on the surface of the T cell into the contact area between the T cell and the antigen presenting cell. This increased local concentration leads to tyrosine phosphorylation of Immunoreceptor Tyrosine-based Activation Motifs (ITAMs) on the cytoplasmic tails of several of the CD3 chains. This in turn recruits further tyrosine kinases (e.g. *zap*), and full-scale activation of the intracellular signalling pathway. Ultimately, these intracellular signals lead to activation of transcription factors, proteins which bind specific sites on DNA and hence regulate transcription of particular sets of genes. One key step in T cells is the activation of the transcription factor NF-AT, and it is this step which is inhibited by cyclosporin, an important immunosuppressant used clinically to block transplant rejection (see Fig. 37).

IL2 One of the main events which follow recognition of antigen by T cells is that the responding T cells undergo several rounds of cell division (a phenomenon known as clonal expansion). T cell proliferation is driven largely by the secretion from the T cells themselves of the cytokine interleukin 2. IL-2 was one of the first of the family of **cytokines** to be identified. As well as its major role in inducing T cell proliferation, it has effects on B lymphocytes, macrophages, eosinophils, etc. (see Fig. 23). T cell activation also results in secretion of many other cytokines, including IFNγ and other cytokines involved in activating macrophages, and IL4, IL5 and IL6 involved mainly in helping B cells make antibody of various different subclasses. The decision as to which sets of cytokines to make is regulated, at least in part, by selective activation of members of the STAT family of transcription factors.

Superantigens There is one exception to the very high specificity of T cell-peptide–MHC interactions: certain molecules, for example some viruses and staphylococcal enterotoxins, have the curious ability to bind to both MHC Class II and the TCR β chain, *outside* the peptide-binding site. The result is that a whole 'family' of T cells respond, rather than a single clone, with excessive and potentially damaging over-production of cytokines.

15 Antibody diversification and synthesis

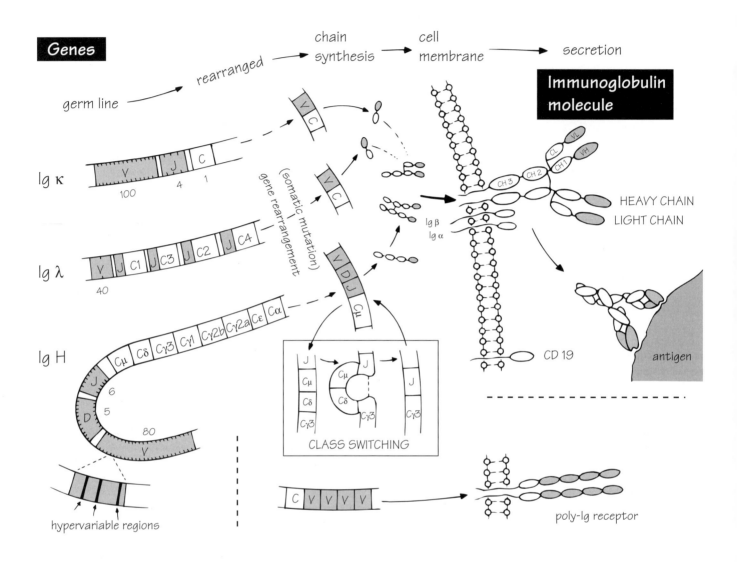

In contrast to the MHC and the T cell receptor, the existence of the antibody, or **immunoglobulin** (Ig) molecule has been known for 100 years and its basic structure for about 30, which makes it one of the most studied and best understood molecules in biology.

The two-chain multidomain structure characteristic of MHC and T cell receptors is seen here in a slightly more complex form, a typical Ig molecule being made up of four chains—a pair of **heavy** chains and a pair of **light chains** (see Fig. 16 for structural details). Two main kinds of diversity are found within these chains: in the **constant** regions of the heavy chains are the variations which classify Ig molecules into classes and subclasses with different biological effects, while the much more

extensive variations in the **variable** regions (shaded in the figure) are responsible for the shape of the antigen-binding site and thus of the antigen specificity of the Ig molecule.

Within B lymphocytes, the genes for Ig heavy and light chains are put together by a process of rearrangement at the DNA level followed by further excisions in the messenger RNA, very much as in T cells with their receptor, one important difference being that in B, but not T, cells, further **somatic mutation** in the variable regions can occur. Finally, the polypeptide chains are synthesized on ribosomes like other proteins, assembled and exported—some to reside on the cell surface as receptors and others to be secreted into the blood as **antibody**.

Ig Immunoglobulin; the name given to all globulins with antibody activity. It has replaced the old term 'gamma globulin' because not all antibodies have gamma electrophoretic mobility.

Igκ, Igλ, IgH Three genetic loci on different chromosomes which code for the light chain (κ, λ) and heavy chain (H) of the Ig molecule. A typical Ig molecule has two H chains and two L chains — either both κ or both λ.

Germ line This denotes those genes in the ova and sperm giving rise to successive generations, which can be regarded as a continuous family tree stretching back to the earliest forms of life. Mutations and other genetic changes in these genes are passed to subsequent generations and are what natural selection works on. Changes which occur in any other cells of the body are 'somatic' and affect only the individual, being lost when he dies. This includes the changes in the DNA of B lymphocytes which lead to the formation of the Ig molecule. The antibody germ line genes have presumably been selected as indispensable, and many of them have been shown to code for antibodies against common bacteria, confirming that bacterial infection was probably the main stimulus for the evolution of antibody.

V Variable region genes. Their number ranges from two (mouse λ chain) to about 350 (mouse κ chain; the numbers shown in the figure are for the human). The greatest variation is found in three short **hypervariable** regions, which code for the amino acids which form the combining site and make contact with the antigen. V genes are classified into **families** on the basis of overall sequence similarity.

C Constant region genes. In the light chains, these code for a single domain only, but in the heavy chains there are three or four domains, numbered CH 1, 2, 3 (4). Which of the eight (mouse) or nine (human) C genes is in use by a particular B lymphocyte determines the class and subclass of the resulting Ig molecule (IgM, IgG, etc., see Fig. 16).

J Joining region genes, coding for the short J segment. Note that in the κ and H chains, the different J genes lie together while in the λ chain each C gene has its own. In primitive vertebrates there are repeated V–J–C segments, which restricts the number of possible combinations.

D Region genes are found only on IgH, where they provide additional possibilities for hypervariability.

Gene rearrangement occurs in the Ig genes of B lymphocytes in a similar way to the TCR genes of T lymphocytes. First the intervening segments of DNA ('introns') between the V and J (and D if present) genes are excised in such a way as to bring together one particular V and one J gene. This is then transcribed to RNA and the segment between this V(D) J segment and the C region are excised (spliced out), to leave an mRNA able to code for a complete V(D) JC chain. This unique process of DNA rearrangements is catalysed by a complex of enzymes many of which are involved in DNA repair functions in other cells. However, the first cleavage of DNA which initiates the recombination event is catalysed by two specialized enzymes RAG-1 and RAG-2 (recombination activating genes) enzymes. These enzymes are expressed only in developing B and T cells, and knocking out these genes in mice results in a complete absence of B or T cells.

Class switching can occur within the individual B cell by further excisions of DNA which allow the same VDJ segment to lie next to a different C gene, leading to antibodies with the same specificity for antigen but a different constant region (see Fig. 16). This allows the same antigen to be subjected to various different forms of attack. The decision which class or subclass to switch to is largely regulated by cytokines released locally by helper T cells; thus IL-4 favours IgE, IL-5 IgA, IFNγ IgG3, etc. (these examples are from the mouse).

CD 19 One of the molecules (the complement receptor CR2 is another) that need to be bound in order to fully activate the B cell, thus playing a 'coreceptor' role somewhat analogous to CD4, CD8 and CD28 on the T cell. CD19 is also a convenient 'marker' for B cells, since it is not expressed on other types of cell.

Origins of diversity Four features of antibody contribute to the enormous number of possible antigen-binding sites, and thus of antibody specificities: (1) gene rearrangement allows any V, D and J genes to become associated; (2) a heavy chain can pair with either a κ or λ light chain; (3) V-D and D-J joining is not always at precisely the same point; (4) mutations can occasionally occur in the V genes of an individual B cell (this would be a case of **somatic mutation**) and the resulting small change in the antigen-binding site may sometimes prove advantageous, for example by increasing the affinity of an antibody for the inducing antigen. Because of all these possibilities it is difficult to put a number on the size of the Ig repertoire, but it probably exceeds 10^8. Note that diversity within the MHC is generated in a quite different way, individuals having only one or two of the allelic variants of each gene. Thus the members of a species differ from each other much more in their MHC genes and molecules than in their Ig and T cell receptors, of which they all have a fairly complete set with only minor inherited differences.

Igα, Igβ Two molecules that form a link between cell-surface Ig and intracellular signalling pathways, analogous to CD3 on the T cell.

16 Antibody structure and function

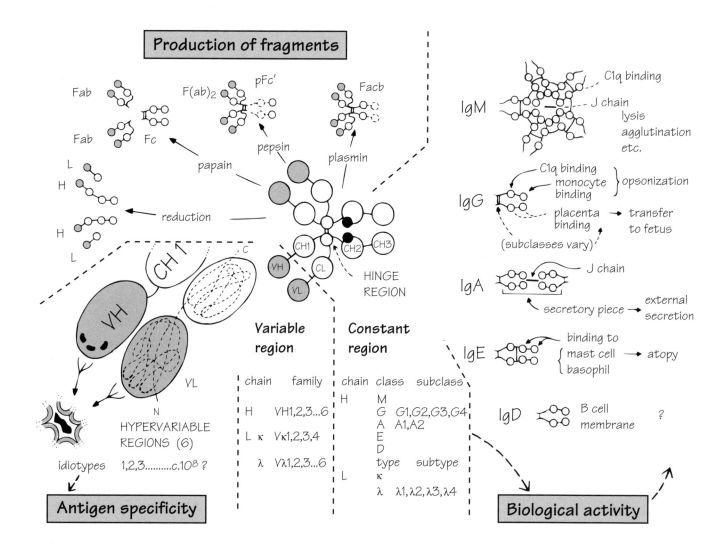

Production of fragments

Fab F(ab)₂ pFc′ Facb

Fab Fc

L
H

H
L

papain pepsin plasmin reduction

CH1 C CH1 VH CL VL CH2 CH3 HINGE REGION

VH VL

N
HYPERVARIABLE REGIONS (6)

idiotypes 1,2,3.........c.10⁸ ?

Antigen specificity

Variable region		Constant region		
chain	family	chain	class	subclass
H	VH1,2,3...6	H	M	
L κ	Vκ1,2,3,4		G	G1,G2,G3,G4
			A	A1,A2
			E	
λ	Vλ1,2,3...6		D	
			type	subtype
		L	κ	
			λ	λ1,λ2,λ3,λ4

IgM — C1q binding — J chain lysis agglutination etc.

IgG — C1q binding — monocyte binding } opsonization — placenta binding → transfer to fetus
(subclasses vary)

IgA — J chain — secretory piece → external secretion

IgE — binding to { mast cell → atopy basophil

IgD — B cell membrane ?

Biological activity

Considering that the antibody in serum is a mixture of perhaps 100 million slightly different types of molecule, the unravelling of its structure was no mean feat. Early work depended on separation into fragments by chemical treatment (top left in figure); the fine details have come from amino acid sequencing and X-ray crystallography, both of which require the use of completely homogeneous (monoclonal) antibody. This was originally available only in the form of myeloma proteins, the product of malignant B lymphocytes, but is produced nowadays by the hybridoma method (see Fig. 9).

A typical antibody molecule (IgG, centre) has 12 domains, arranged in two heavy and two light (H and L) chains, linked through cysteine residues by disulphide bonds so that the domains lie together in pairs, the whole molecule having the shape of a flexible **Y**. In each chain the N-terminal domain is the most **variable**, the rest being relatively **constant**. Within the variable (V) regions, the maximum variation in amino acid sequence is seen in the six **hypervariable** regions (three per chain) which come together to form the **antigen-binding site** (bottom left in

figure). The constant (C) regions vary mainly in those portions which interact with complement or various cell-surface receptors; the right-hand part of the figure shows the different features of the C region in the five **classes** of antibody; M, G, A, E and D. The result is a huge variety of molecules able to bring any antigen into contact with any one of several effective disposal mechanisms. The basic structure (MW, about 160 000) can form dimers (IgA, MW 400 000) or pentamers (IgM, MW 900 000; see right-hand side of figure).

There are species differences, especially in the heavy chain subclasses, which have evolved comparatively recently; the examples shown here illustrate human antibodies. Attention has recently been focused on the carbohydrate side chains (show here in black) which may constitute up to 12% of the whole molecule. They are thought to be associated mainly with secretion, but are abnormal in certain diseases.

Note The illustration shows an IgG molecule with its 12 domains stylized. The actual 3-dimensional structure is more like the molecule shown binding to antigen in Fig. 15 (extreme right).

Fragments produced by chemical treatment:
• H, L: Heavy and light chains which, being only disulphide-linked, separate under reducing conditions.
• Fab: antigen-binding fragment (papain digestion).
• Fc: crystallizable (because relatively homogeneous fragment) (papain digestion).
• F(ab)₂: two Fab fragments united by disulphide bonds (pepsin digestion).
• pFc′: a dimer of CH3 domains (pepsin digestion).
• Facb: an Ig molecule lacking CH3 domains (plasmin digestion).

Chains   The heavy and two types of light (κ, λ) chains are coded for by genes on different chromosomes, but sequence homologies suggest that all Ig domains originated from a common 'precursor' molecule about 110 amino acids long (see Fig. 12).

Classes   Physical, antigenic and functional variations between constant regions define the five main classes of heavy chain: M, G, A, E and D. These are different molecules, all of which are present in all members of most higher species. Brief points of interest are listed below.

IgM is usually the first class of antibody made in a response and is also thought to have been the first to appear during evolution (see Fig. 3). Because its pentameric structure gives it up to 10 antigen-combining sites, it is extremely efficient at binding and agglutinating micro-organisms.

IgG, a later development which owes its value to the ability of its Fc portion to bind avidly to C1q (see Fig. 5) and to receptors on phagocytic cells (see Fig. 8). It also gains access to the extravascular spaces and (via the placenta) to the fetus. In most species, IgG has become further diversified into subclasses (see below).

IgA is the major antibody of secretions such as tears, sweat and the contents of lungs, gut, urine, etc., where, thanks to its secretory piece (see below), it avoids digestion. Its main value is to block the entry of micro-organisms from these external surfaces to the tissues themselves.

IgE is a curious molecule whose main property is to bind to mast cells and promote their degranulation. The desirable and undesirable consequences of this are discussed in Fig. 33.

IgD appears to function only on the surface of B cells, where it may have some regulatory role. In the mouse it is unusual in having two instead of three constant regions in the heavy chain.

Subclasses, subtypes   Within classes, smaller variations between constant regions define the subclasses found in different molecules of all members of an individual species. The IgG subclasses are generally the most varied. Light chain C region variants of this kind are sometimes called 'subtypes'. All these variants found in all individuals of a species are called 'isotypic'. Different IgG subclasses tend to be induced by different types of antigen (e.g. in man, IgG1 and 3 by viruses, IgG2 by carbohydrates) but nobody really knows why this is.

Allotypes   By contrast, 'allotypic' variations (not shown in the figure) distinguish the Ig molecules of some individuals from others (cf. the blood groups). They are genetically determined or perhaps regulated, and occur mainly in the C regions. No biological function has yet been discovered. Unlike blood groups, etc., Ig allotypes are expressed singly on individual B cells, a process known as 'allelic exclusion', which shows that only one of the cell's two sets of chromosomes are used for making antibody—presumably the first one to successfully rearrange its Ig genes.

Hypervariable regions   Three parts of each of the variable regions of heavy and light chains, spaced roughly equally apart in the amino acid sequence (see figure, lower left) but brought close together as the chain folds into a β-pleated sheet, form the antigen-combining site. It is because of the enormous degree of variation in the DNA coding for these regions that the total number of combinations is so high. The hypervariable regions are also unusually susceptible to further **somatic mutation**, which occurs during B cell proliferation within the germinal centre of lymph nodes or spleen. This further increases the range of available combining sites.

Idiotypes   In many cases, antibody molecules with different antigen-combining sites can in turn be distinguished by other antibodies made against them. The latter are known as 'anti-idiotypic', implying that each combining site is associated with a different shape, though this is not always the antigen-binding site itself. Anti-idiotypic antibodies are thought to be formed normally and may help to regulate immune responses (see Fig. 22).

Hinge region   Both flexibility and proteolytic digestion are facilitated by the repeated proline residues in this part of the molecule. In IgM, the hinge region is as large as a normal domain, and is called CH2, so that the other two constant region domains are called CH3 and CH4; the same may be true for IgE.

J chain   A glycopeptide molecule which aids polymerization of IgA and IgM.

Secretory piece   A polypeptide derived from the Poly Ig receptor (see Fig. 15) and added to IgA dimers in epithelial cells to enable them to be transported across the epithelium and secreted into the gut, tears, milk, etc. where IgA predominates.

C1q   The first component of the classical complement sequence, a hexavalent glycoprotein activated by binding to CH2 domains of IgM and some IgG subclasses (in the human, IgG1 and IgG3; see also Fig. 5).

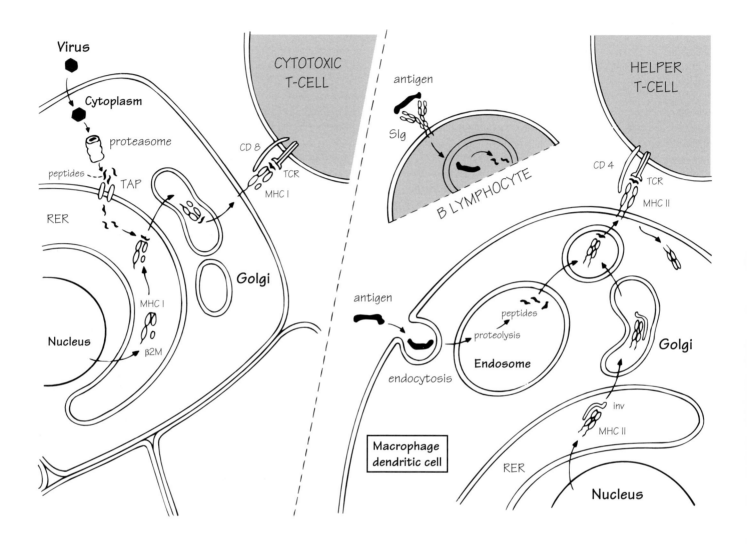

In discussing the MHC and the T cell receptor (Figs 13, 14), frequent allusion has been made to the foreign peptides which bind to the former and are recognized by the latter. The discovery of how these peptides are produced and how they become associated with MHC molecules has been one of the triumphs of recent immunology. In the figure are shown the two quite separate pathways, usually known for convenience as the 'Class I pathway' (left) and the 'Class II pathway' (right).

The first evidence that the MHC was involved in presenting antigens to T cells was the demonstration of '**MHC restriction**' —the fact that T cells are specific for both antigen and MHC molecule. Then it was discovered that cytotoxic T cells could respond to viral nuclear antigens, which are not displayed on the surface of the virus! How could a T cell 'see' such a well-concealed antigen? The answer is shown in the left-hand figure above: virus-derived peptides become bound to Class I MHC molecules inside the cell and are then transported to the surface, where T cells can recognize the peptide-MHC combination and, under

appropriate circumstances, kill the virus-infected cell (see Fig. 20 for more details).

At the same time, it was shown that a rather similar process occurs in the 'antigen-presenting' cells, mainly macrophages and dendritic cells, which activate helper T cells —with the difference that here it is the Class II MHC molecules that transport the peptides to the surface (right-hand figure). This process is kept separate from the Class I pathway by occurring in the endosomal/lysosomal vacuoles in which foreign material is normally digested (see Fig. 8). More recently, it was shown that B lymphocytes, as well as receiving T-cell help, could also process and present antigen, but only when they were able to bind it via their surface immunoglobulin (see Fig. 18).

One can now appreciate that the real role of the MHC system is to transport samples of **intracellular proteins** to the cell surface for T cells to inspect them and react if necessary —by proliferating into clones and then helping macrophages or B cells or killing virus-infected cells, as described in the following pages.

The class I pathway

Virus Since they are synthesized in the cell, viral proteins are available in the cytoplasm, alongside self-proteins.

RER Rough endoplasmic reticulum, where proteins, including those of the MHC, are synthesized.

MHC I The single 3-domain α chain associates with **β2 microglobulin** to make a Class I MHC molecule, whose structure is not fully stable until a peptide has been bound (see below).

Proteasome A cylindrical complex of proteolytic enzymes with the property of digesting proteins into short peptides. Two components of the proteasome are encoded by the LMP genes which are found within the MHC region of the chromosome.

TAP TAP (transporter of antigen peptide) genes are found within MHC region of the chromosome, and encode transporter proteins which carry the proteolytic fragments of antigen generated by the proteasome from the cytosol into the lumen of the endoplasmic reticulum where they bind to the peptide-binding groove of the class I MHC.

Peptides of 8–10 amino acids are able to bind into the groove between the first two α chains of the MHC molecule, mainly by their terminal amino acids. This binding is of high affinity but not as specific as that of antibody or the TCR. Thus the six different types of Class I MHC molecules on each cell (see Fig. 13), can between them bind a wide range of peptides, including many derived from 'self' proteins. Most of the peptides bound to MHC at any one time will be derived from 'self' proteins from within the cell. Even after viral infection only a few percent of the available MHC molecules become loaded with viral peptides.

Golgi The Golgi complex, responsible for conveying proteins from the RER to other sites, including the cell surface. Once on the surface, the MHC-peptide combination is available to interact with an appropriate T cell.

TCR The T cell receptor. Because of selection in the thymus (see Fig. 10), only a T cell whose receptor recognizes both the MHC molecule and the peptide bound in it, will respond. This is a highly specific interaction, ensuring that cells displaying only 'self' peptides are not killed.

CD8 This molecule, expressed on cytotoxic T cells, recognizes the Class I MHC molecule, a further requirement before killing of the virus-infected cell by the **cytotoxic T cell** can take place.

The class II pathway

Antigen Any foreign material taken in by phagocytosis or endocytosis will find itself in vesicles of the endocytic pathway, collectively known as **endosomes**, but including the acidic lysosomes, so that various digestive enzymes can act at the appropriate pH. In the case of microbial infection, it will be the whole microbe that is taken in.

SIg Surface immunoglobulin allows the B lymphocyte to bind and subsequently endocytose antigen.

MHC II The two-chain MHC Class II molecule forms a peptide-binding groove between the α1 and β1 domains, the β chain contributing most of the specificity. When first synthesized, this binding is prevented by a protein called the **invariant chain**, which is progressively cleaved off and replaced by newly produced peptides in the endosomes.

Inv (Invariant chain). So called because, in contrast to the Class II MHC molecules, it is not polymorphic. This molecule performs a number of important functions in the Class II processing pathway. It acts as a 'chaperone' in helping MHC molecules to fold correctly as they are synthesized, and then binds to them, preventing peptides from associating with the peptide-binding site while still within the endoplasmic reticulum. It then directs the transport of the associated Class II MHC molecules to specialized processing endosomes where, finally, it is proteolytically cleaved. This allows antigen peptides to bind the MHC, and allows the MHC carrying the peptides to exit the endosome and go to the cell membrane.

Peptides MHC Class II molecules can bind peptides up to 20 amino acids long—longer than Class I MHC since the MHC Class II peptide binding groove allows peptides to extend out of each end. The peptides include some derived from microbes in the endosomes (e.g. persistent bacteria such as TB), but also includes many self-peptides, many of which are derived from MHC molecules themselves. The binding of peptides to MHC is facilitated and regulated by two other Class II-like molecules HLA-DM and HLA-DO which are also found within the processing endosome.

CD4 This molecule, expressed on **helper T cells**, interacts with MHC Class II molecules, ensuring that the T cell response (i.e. cytokine secretion; see Fig. 18) is focused on an appropriate cell—that is, either a B lymphocyte or a macrophage harbouring an intracellular infection.

Thus the type of T cell response that occurs is determined by a sequence of factors, namely: (i) the type of T cell—CD8 cytotoxic or CD4 helper; (ii) the class of MHC—I or II; (iii) the source of the peptide bound by the MHC—cytoplasmic or endocytosed; and ultimately (iv) the type of infection—viral or microbial. However, there are exceptions to this tidy scheme, as described in Figs 26–29.

18 The antibody response

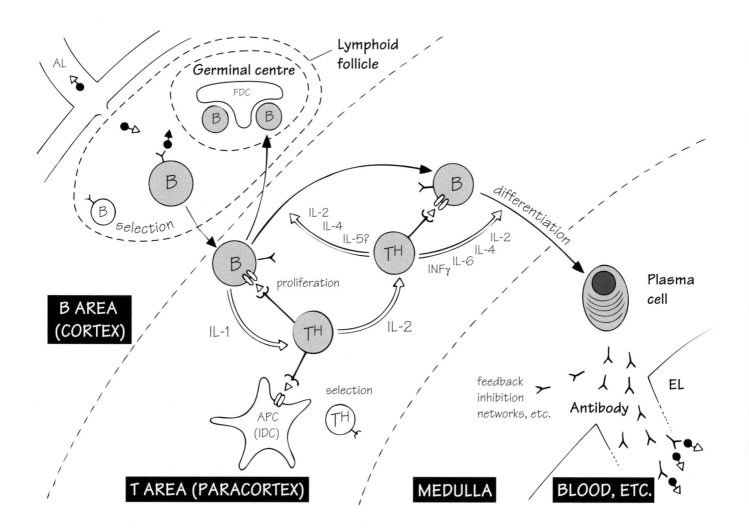

Animals born and reared in the complete absence of contact with any non-self material (not an easy procedure!) have virtually no immunoglobulins in their serum, but as soon as they encounter the normal environment, with its content of bacteria, etc., their serum immunoglobulin (Ig) rises towards the normal level of 10–20 mg (or about 60 000 000 000 000 000 molecules) per ml. This shows that immunoglobulins are produced only as a result of stimulation by foreign antigens, the process being known as the **antibody response**.

In the figure, these events are shown in a section through a stylized lymph node. Antigen is shown entering from the tissues (top left) and antibody being released into the blood (bottom right). The antigen is depicted as a combination of two components, representing the portion, or **determinant**, recognized by the B cell and against which antibody is eventually made (black circles) and other determinants which interact with T cells and are needed in order for the B cell to be fully triggered (white triangles). These are usually known as '**haptenic**' and '**carrier**' determinants, respectively. In practice, a virus, bacterium, etc. would carry numerous different haptenic and carrier determinants, whereas small molecules such as toxins may act as haptens only. But even small,

well-defined antigenic determinants usually stimulate a heterogeneous population of B cells, each producing antibody of slightly different specificity and affinity.

The main stages of the response are recognition and **processing** of the antigen (see Fig. 17), **selection** of the appropriate individual B and T cells (shown shaded), **proliferation** of these cells to form a **clone** and **differentiation** into the mature **functioning** state. A prominent feature of all stages is the many **interactions** between cells which are mediated mostly by cytokines (white arrows in the figure). There are also a number of regulatory influences whose relative importance is not yet clear. Most of these cell interactions occur in the lymph nodes or spleen, but antibody can be formed wherever there is lymphoid tissue.

In a subsequent response to the same antigen, average affinity tends to be higher, precursor T and B cells more numerous and Ig class more varied. This **secondary** response is therefore more rapid and effective, and such an individual is described as showing **memory** to the antigen in question; this, for example, is the aim of most vaccines (see Fig. 41).

AL Afferent lymphatic, via which antigens and antigen-bearing cells enter the lymph node from the tissues (see Fig. 11).

APC Antigen-presenting cell. Before they can trigger lymphocytes, antigens normally require to be presented on the surface of a specialized cell. This function is performed for B cells by follicular dendritic cells (FDC), and for T cells by interdigitating dendritic cells (IDC). Various dendritic cells in lymphoid tissue, Langerhans cells in the skin, etc. (see Fig. 7) can perform this function, part of which consists of releasing Interleukin-1 (IL-1) (see below) but which in the case of T lymphocytes also requires the presence of Class II MHC molecules on the APC. Except with small peptides that can associate directly with MHC, antigens have to be **processed** first (see Fig. 17, right-hand side, for an enlarged version of this stage).

FDC The follicular dendritic cell, specialized for presenting antigen to B lymphocytes in the B cell follicles. Antigen on the surface of FDC is largely intact, maintaining its native conformation, and is often held in the form of antibody/antigen complexes which can persist for weeks or months.

IDC The interdigitating dendritic cell, specialized for presenting peptides to T cells in the T cell area or paracortex. This cell is derived from 'immature' dendritic cells found within most tissues of the body (those in skin, for example, are known as Langerhans cells) which take up antigen by pinocytosis or phagocytosis, process it (see Fig. 17) and then migrate through the afferent lymphatics to the nearest lymph node. IDC express very high levels of MHC on the cell surface, as well as a variety of ligands for T cell costimulatory molecules (see Fig. 14).

Selection Only a small minority of lymphocytes will recognize and bind to a particular antigen. These lymphocytes are thus 'selected' by the antigen. The binding 'receptor' is surface Ig in the case of the B cell, and the TCR complex in the case of the T cell, which recognizes both antigen and MHC (see Figs 14, 17).

Clonal proliferation Once selected, lymphocytes divide repeatedly to form a 'clone' of identical cells. The stimuli for B cell proliferation are a variety of T cell-derived cytokines and adhesion molecule interactions (see Fig. 14). T cell proliferation is greatly augmented by another soluble factor (**IL-2**) made by T cells themselves. (For more information on interleukins see Fig. 23). The combination of selection by antigen followed by clonal proliferation has given to the whole lymphocyte response the descriptive name of **clonal selection**.

Differentiation Once they have proliferated, B cells become susceptible to helper factors from T helper (T^H) cells. Those that have been identified have been given 'interleukin' numbers but almost all the known cytokines have some effect in promoting B cell growth or function. However, certain large repeating antigens can do this without T cell help; they are called 'T independent' and are usually bacterial polysaccharides. As a rule they only stimulate IgM, probably representing a more primitive form of response.

Plasma cell In order to make and secrete antibody, endoplasmic reticulum and ribosomes are developed, giving the B cell its basophilic excentric appearance. Plasma cells can release up to 2000 antibody molecules per second, but they only live for a few days.

EL Efferent lymphatic, via which antibody formed in the medulla reaches the lymph and eventually the blood for distribution to all parts of the body.

Memory cells Instead of differentiating into antibody-producing plasma cells, some B cells persist as memory cells, whose increased number and rapid response underlies the highly augmented secondary response, essentially a faster and larger version of the primary response, starting out from more of the appropriate B (and T^H) cells. Memory B cells differ slightly from their precursors (more surface Ig, more likely to recirculate in the blood) but retain the same specificity for antigen. The generation of memory B cells appears to take place in **germinal centres** and to require the presence of complement. It is also somehow linked to T cells, since T independent responses do not usually show memory. T^H cells also develop into memory cells but their precise location is not known. Exactly how long individual memory cells survive and whether they need repeated restimulation is still controversial.

Feedback inhibition Antibody itself, particularly IgG, can inhibit its own formation, either by eliminating the antigen or by preventing it stimulating B cells. T cells which suppress antibody production have also been described (T^S). Although these cells have still not been fully characterized (see Fig. 21), they always act by regulating the T^H cell, rather than by directly suppressing the B cell itself.

Networks It was hypothesized by Jerne, and subsequently shown, that antibody idiotypes (i.e. the unique portions related to specificity) can themselves act as antigens, and promote both B and T cell responses against the cells carrying them, so that the immune response progressively damps itself out. This leads to the fascinating concept of a network of anti-idiotype receptors corresponding to all the antigens an animal can respond to—a sort of 'internal image' of its external environment (see Fig. 22 for a further discussion). However, the actual role of networks in regulating ordinary antibody responses is not yet clear, nor is that of suppressor T cells. In practice the single most important element in regulating antibody production is probably the removal of the antigen itself.

19 Antigen–antibody interaction and immune complexes

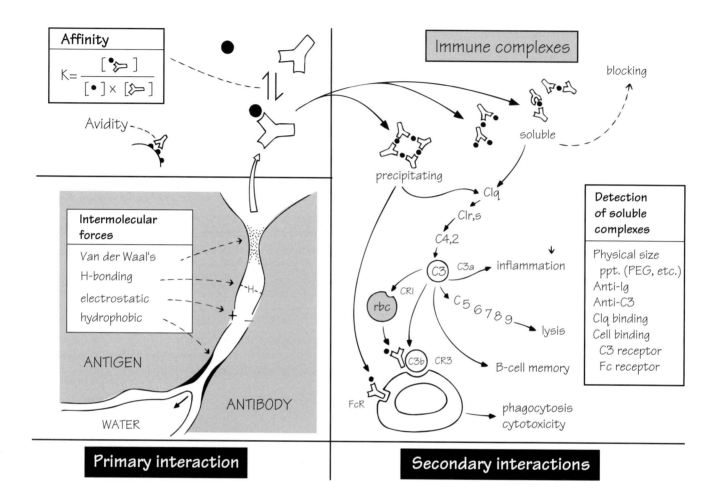

Primary interaction

Affinity
$$K = \frac{[\,\bullet\!\!-\!\!\diamond\,]}{[\,\bullet\,] \times [\,\diamond\,]}$$

Avidity

Intermolecular forces
- Van der Waal's
- H-bonding
- electrostatic
- hydrophobic

ANTIGEN

ANTIBODY

WATER

Secondary interactions

Immune complexes

blocking

soluble

precipitating

C1q

C1r,s

C4,2

C3 — C3a — inflammation

CR1

rbc

C 5 6 7 8 9 — lysis

C3b CR3 — B-cell memory

FcR — phagocytosis cytotoxicity

Detection of soluble complexes
- Physical size ppt. (PEG, etc.)
- Anti-Ig
- Anti-C3
- C1q binding
- Cell binding
  - C3 receptor
  - Fc receptor

An antigen, by definition, stimulates the production of antibody, which in turn combines with the antigen. Both processes are based on **complementarity** (or 'fit') between two **shapes**—a small piece of the antigen (or **determinant**) and the **combining site** of the antibody, a cleft formed largely by the hypervariable regions of heavy and light chains (see Fig. 16). The closer the fit between this site and the antigenic determinant, the stronger will be the non-covalent forces (hydrophobic, electrostatic, etc., lower left) between them, and the higher the **affinity** (top left). When both combining sites can interact with the same antigen (e.g. on a cell), the bond has a greatly increased strength, which in this case is referred to as 'avidity'.

The ability of a particular antibody to combine with one determinant rather than another is referred to as **specificity**. The antibody repertoire of an animal, stored in its V genes and expanded further by mutation (see Fig. 15), is expressed as the number of different shapes towards which a complementary specific antibody molecule can be made, and runs into millions.

What happens when antigen and antibody combine depends on the circumstances. Sometimes antibody alone is enough to neutralize the antigen, as in the case of those toxins or micro-organisms which need to attach to cell surface receptors in order to gain entry; antibody can often block this.

Usually, however, a secondary interaction of the antibody molecule with another effector agent, such as complement or phagocytic cells, is required to dispose of the antigen. The importance of these secondary interactions is shown by the fact that deficiency of complement or myeloid cells can be almost as serious as deficiency of antibody itself (see Fig. 39).

The combination of antigen and antibody is called an **immune complex**; this may be small (soluble) or large (precipitating), depending on the nature and proportions of antigen and antibody (top right). The usual fate of complexes is to be removed by phagocytic cells, through the interaction of the Fc portion of the antibody with complement and with cell-surface receptors (bottom centre and Fig. 8). However, in some cases complexes may persist in circulation and cause inflammatory damage to organs (see Fig. 34) or inhibit useful immunity, for example to tumours or parasites. The detection of complexes and the identification of the antigen in them is therefore important and numerous techniques are available.

Antigen–antibody interaction

The combining site of antibody is a cleft roughly $3 \times 1 \times 1$ nm (the size of five or six sugar units), though there is evidence that antigens may bind to larger, or even separate, parts of the variable region. Binding depends on a close 3-dimensional fit, allowing weak intermolecular forces to overcome the normal repulsion between molecules.

Van der Waal's forces attract all molecules through their electron clouds, but only act at extremely close range.

Hydrogen bonding (e.g. between -NH_2 and -OH groups) is another weak force.

Electrostatic attraction between antibody and antigen molecules with a net opposite charge is sometimes quite strong.

Hydrophobic regions on antigen and antibody will tend to be attracted in an aqueous environment; this is probably the strongest force between them.

Affinity is normally expressed as the association constant under equilibrium conditions. A value of 10^3 litres/mole would be considered low, while high affinity antibody can reach 10^{10} litres/mole and over—several orders of magnitude higher than most enzyme–substrate interactions. In practice, it is often **avidity** which is measured because antibodies have (at least) two valencies, and even with monovalent antigens a serum can only be assigned an average affinity. Average affinity tends to increase with time after antigenic stimulation, partly through cell selection by diminishing amounts of antigen, and partly via somatic mutation of Ig genes. High affinity antibodies are more effective in most cases, but low affinity antibodies persist too, and may have certain advantages (re-usability, resistance to tolerance?).

Immune complexes

Under conditions of antigen or antibody excess, small ('soluble') complexes tend to predominate, but with roughly equivalent amounts of antigen and antibody, precipitates form, probably by lattice formation. In the presence of complement (i.e. in fresh serum) only small complexes are formed; in fact C3 can actually solubilize larger complexes (see also Fig. 34).

Blocking of T cell or antibody-mediated killing by complexes in (respectively) antigen or antibody excess, may account for some of the unresponsiveness to tumours or parasite infections.

C1q the first component of complement, binds to the Fc portion of complexed antibody, possibly under the influence of a conformational change in the shape of the Ig molecule, although some workers hold that occupation of both combining sites (i.e. of IgG) is all that is needed. Activation of the 'classical' complement pathway follows.

Inflammation Breakdown products of C3 and C5, through interaction with mast cells, polymorphs, etc., are responsible for the vascular damage which is a feature of 'immune complex diseases' (see Fig. 34).

Lysis (e.g. of bacteria) requires the complete complement sequence. Sometimes the C567 unit moves away from the original site of antibody binding, activates C8 and 9, and causes lysis of innocent cells (e.g. red cells); this is known as 'reactive lysis'.

Phagocytosis by macrophages, polymorphs, eosinophils, etc. is the normal fate of large complexes. In general, the antibody classes and subclasses which bind to Fc receptors also bind to complement, making them strongly opsonic, but the Fc and C3 receptors are quite distinct; IgM, for example, binds to complement much more than to cells. The majority of complexes in the circulation are picked up by red blood cells (**rbc** in figure) via their complement receptors (see Fig. 5). In transit through the liver and spleen, the complexes are removed by phagocytic cells.

Cytotoxicity When antibody bound to a cell or micro-organism makes contact with Fc receptors, the result may be killing rather than phagocytosis. Cells able to do this include macrophages, monocytes, neutrophils, eosinophils, and the lymphocyte-like 'K' cell (see Fig. 9). The importance of this type of 'antibody-mediated cytotoxicity' *in vivo* is controversial.

B cell memory Complement receptors on the follicular dendritic cells (see Fig. 18) help them to retain immune complexes and present the antigen to B cells in a way that, by selecting for mutants with high binding affinity, encourages the increase or 'maturation' of the antibody response as a whole.

Detection of soluble complexes
Complexes tend to be of large size (e.g. in the ultracentrifuge or gradients), and to precipitate in the cold ('cryoprecipitation') and in polyethylene glycol (PEG). Since they contain Ig, complexes react with anti-Ig antibodies (e.g. rheumatoid factor). Their reaction with C1q is used in a number of sensitive assays, and the presence of C3 can be deduced from reaction with anti-C3 antibody (immunoconglutinin) and binding to cells with C3 receptors, such as the Raji cell line. In general, these assays agree, but some complexes do not fix complement yet are precipitated by PEG, while some tests can be complicated by the presence of other large molecules. Therefore several tests may need to be done in parallel.

20 Cell-mediated immune responses

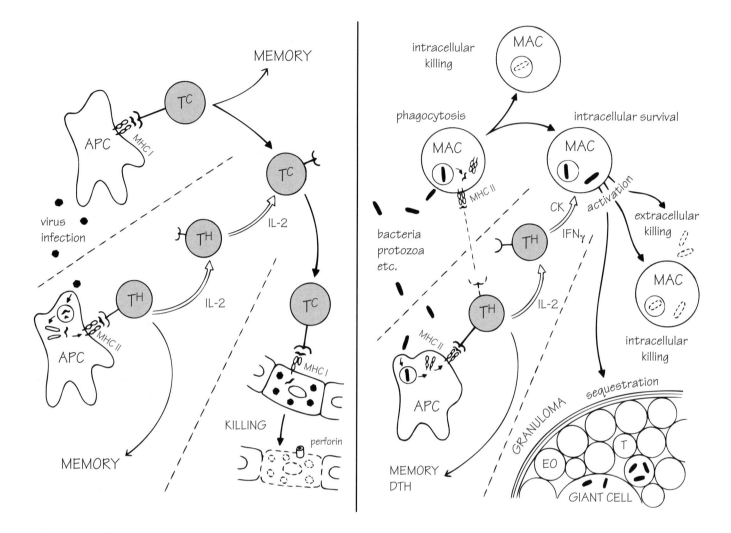

Not all adaptive immunity involves antibody; there is a very important group of responses mediated by T lymphocytes, and showing the characteristic adaptive features of specificity and memory, in which B lymphocytes play no part. Originally identified by their role in immunity to tuberculosis and later found to be also involved in contact sensitivity, immunity to viruses, graft rejection, chronic inflammation and tumour immunity, these responses are usually lumped together under the term 'cell-mediated immunity' (CMI). This is rather misleading because it covers at least two quite different responses: the generation of specific **cytotoxic T cells** against intracellular viruses (left half of figure) and the effect of T cells in increasing the activities of 'non-specific' cells such as macrophages, generally to enable them to deal more vigorously with intracellular bacteria and other parasites (right half of figure). Even more confusingly, this latter type of response is often referred to as **delayed hypersensitivity**, which really only describes a particular kind of skin test used to measure it.

These responses do, however, share many features in common with the antibody response, namely interactions involving T helper cells and antigen presentation in association with products of the MHC (see Figs 13, 14, 17). The way in which these fundamentally useful responses can be a nuisance by causing tissue damage and the rejection of grafts is described in Figs 35 and 37, respectively.

Like the antibody response, too, cell-mediated immunity is regulated by various suppressor cells and factors (not shown in the figure) whose normal function is presumably to limit damaging side-effects but which in some diseases seriously impair the proper protective working of the system.

Viruses cannot survive for long outside the cells of the host, which they replicate in, spread from and sometimes destroy (for further details see Fig. 26).

MHC I Class I MHC molecules (A, B, C in man, KDL in mouse, see Fig. 13) which are an essential part of the recognition of viral antigens by the receptor on cytotoxic CD8 T cells. The CD8 molecule also contributes — refer back to Figs 14 and 17 for a reminder of how.

T^C The cytotoxic or 'killer' T cell whose function is the detection and destruction of virus-infected cells. Its receptor recognizes 'self' Class I MHC antigens plus 'non-self' virus antigen, and the latter recognition is highly specific, i.e. there are different T cells for different viruses, which are selected and clonally proliferated like B cells.

APC Although Class I MHC is present on most cell types, thus allowing T^c to recognize and destroy any virally infected cells, T^c have first to be 'primed' by antigen-presenting cells (also known as dendritic cells) carrying viral antigens in association with Class I MHC on their surface. For most antiviral responses, the T^c response is much more effective and long-lived if virus also stimulates CD4 'helper' cells, which recognize viral antigens in association with class II MHC on the antigen presenting cell.

T^H A helper T cell, similar to the T^H for antibody responses, which secretes cytokines (especially IL-2 and IFN$_\gamma$) which cause T^C to proliferate and differentiate into mature killer cells, and macrophages to become activated and kill intracellular pathogens (see T^{H1} and T^{H2} cells, Fig. 9).

IL-2 Interleukin-2, a T cell-derived cytokine. It is a glycoprotein of MW 15500, and varies considerably from species to species. It can only act on cells which have a **receptor** for it, the development of which is an essential part of T cell maturation. IL-2 used to be known as T cell growth factor or TCGF (see also Fig. 23).

Killing Once fully mature, T^C will kill any cell on whose surface they recognize the same combination of Class I MHC antigen plus virus. Killing occurs in two stages: **binding** by the receptor, and a Ca^{2+} dependent **lysis** of the target cell. A key feature of all T cell killing is that it works by activating the target cell to commit suicide, a process known as apoptosis (or programmed cell death). Once initiated this process can continue after the T^C has detached, so that one T^C can kill several target cells. Killing is principally carried out by the secretion of **perforins and granzymes.** Perforins are small pore-forming molecules similar to the terminal complement lytic complex. Insertion of these molecules into the target cell membrane allows the entry of granzymes, proteolytic enzymes which activate the caspase cascade, and thus initiate apoptosis. Some T^c use an alternative pathway, in which Fas-ligand on the T cell (a molecule belonging to the TNF family) interacts with Fas receptor on the target, to initiate apoptosis.

Bacteria Certain bacteria, protozoa and fungi as well as many viruses, having been **phagocytosed** by macrophages (MAC) avoid the normal fate of **intracellular killing** (see Fig. 8 for details) and **survive**, either within the phagolysosome or free in the cytosol. In the absence of assistance from the T cells this would result in progressive and incurable infection. Note that the T helper cells involved here need to secrete IFN$_\gamma$

and other macrophage activating factors in order to function. In current terminology, they would be of the T^{H1} type.

CK Cytokines, a large family of molecules produced by lymphoid and myeloid cells which regulate the activity of both haemopoetic and non-haemopoetic cells. Most cytokines have a very short half-life after they are secreted, so their activity is limited to the immediate environment of the activated cell. This is important because cytokines, once released, do not have any intrinsic antigen specificity. Some of the main CK involved in cellular immunity are (see Fig. 23 for more details):
• IL-2: see above.
• MIF: macrophage migration inhibition factor, which by restricting the movement of macrophages, concentrates them in the vicinity of the T cell.
• MAF: macrophage activating factors, which increase many macrophage functions, including intracellular killing and the secretion of various cytotoxic factors able to kill organisms **extracellularly**.
• Interferon: ('immune' or γ); an important antiviral and regulatory molecule and the major component of MAF.
• Lymphotoxin: possibly important in killing some tumour cells (see Fig. 31 for further details).
• B cell growth factors: see Fig. 18.
• CSF: colony-stimulating factors, stimulatory for monocyte differentiation and perhaps for the secretion of IL-1.
IL-1: an unusual CK, in that it acts systemically through the body, activating the acute phase response in liver (see Fig. 6), and increasing body temperature (fever) via its action on the hypothalamous.
• TNF-α: an important cytokine in the regulation of inflammation, via its effect on the properties of endothelium, causing leucocytes to adhere to the wall of the blood vessel and migrate into tissues. Like IL-1 it can act systemically, and if produced in excess can cause 'wasting', fever and joint destruction.

Granuloma Undegradeable material (e.g. tubercle bacilli, streptococcal cell walls, talc) may be **sequestered** in a focus of concentric macrophages often containing some T cells, eosinophils (EO) and **giant** cells, made from the fusion of several macrophages. For the role of granulomata in chronic inflammation see Fig. 35.

Memory All the T cells involved in CMI can give rise to memory cells and thus secondary responses of increased effectiveness. Note that in the macrophage type of CMI the memory is entirely in the T^H cells. 'Memory' T cells are present with greater frequency than 'naïve' T cells, but are also biochemically distinct in that they can be stimulated by lower doses of antigen. Persistence of memory can apparently occur in the complete absence of antigen, although memory cells continually divide at a slow rate.

DTH Delayed-type hypersensitivity. The first evidence for adaptive immunity in tuberculosis was the demonstration (Koch, 1891) that injection of a tubercle antigen 'tuberculin' into the skin caused a swollen red reaction a day or more later. In patients with antibody, the corresponding reaction would take only hours, whence the terms 'delayed' and 'acute' hypersensitivity, respectively. DTH depends on the presence of T memory cells; the changes shown in the figure (right-hand side) occur at the site of injection, together with increased vascular permeability. Thus DTH is a useful model of normal CMI and also a convenient test for T cell memory.

21 Tolerance

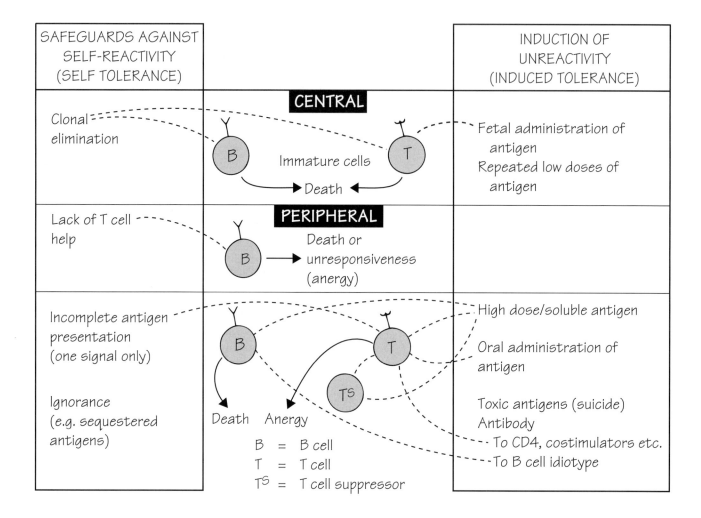

SAFEGUARDS AGAINST SELF-REACTIVITY (SELF TOLERANCE) | INDUCTION OF UNREACTIVITY (INDUCED TOLERANCE)

CENTRAL

Clonal elimination — Immature cells → Death ← — Fetal administration of antigen / Repeated low doses of antigen

PERIPHERAL

Lack of T cell help — Death or unresponsiveness (anergy)

Incomplete antigen presentation (one signal only) — Death / Anergy — High dose/soluble antigen / Oral administration of antigen / Toxic antigens (suicide) / Antibody: To CD4, costimulators etc. / To B cell idiotype

Ignorance (e.g. sequestered antigens)

B = B cell
T = T cell
Tˢ = T cell suppressor

The evolution of recognition systems that initiate destruction of 'non-self' material obviously brings with it the need for safeguards to prevent damage to 'self'. The problem is somewhat different for the natural and adaptive immune systems. Natural mechanisms such as phagocytosis, direct activation of C3, lysozyme, C-reactive protein (CRP), etc., are normally active against only a restricted range of substances exclusive to micro-organisms or to already damaged 'self' material. Adaptive mechanisms—that is, T and B lymphocytes—having evolved a huge range of receptors to fill the gaps in the natural system, must somehow distinguish those which happen to react against shapes found on the animal's other molecules. Such unreactivity cannot be 'built in' genetically, since the receptors and the 'self' molecules they might recognize are inherited quite separately. For example, people of blood group A make antibodies to blood group B and vice versa. Thus the AB child of an A father and a B mother inherits the ability to make both and anti-A antibodies but must not make either: that is, must be **tolerant** to A and B.

Within the lymphoid system, immune responses are in fact protected against self-reactivity at several levels. The central part of the figure depicts the key types of adaptive response, already described in further detail in Figs 18 and 20, while the other panels show the principal safeguards. It used to be assumed that elimination of potentially self-reactive clones was the basis of all unresponsiveness to self, but many other regulatory mechanisms are now recognized. Failure of any one of these may lead to self-destructive immune responses (see Fig. 36). Note also that self-unreactivity 'ignorance' to certain antigens (e.g. lens protein) is due not to the absence of reactive lymphocytes but to the 'sequestration' of the antigens.

In certain circumstances (extreme right), these safeguarding mechanisms can also be triggered by normally antigenic 'non-self' materials in which case these are subsequently treated essentially like 'self', a state known as **tolerance**, which might be very undesirable in some infections but very useful in the case of an organ transplant. Note that tolerance is by definition **antigen-specific**, and quite distinct from the non-specific unresponsiveness induced by damage to the immune system as a whole (see Fig. 38). Note also that in some older books the term 'tolerance' is often restricted to proved cases of clonal elimination; unfortunately clonal elimination is usually rather difficult to prove.

Safeguards against self-reactivity

Clonal elimination A cornerstone of Burnet's Clonal Selection Theory (1959) was the prediction that lymphocytes were individually restricted in their recognition of antigen and that self-recognizing ones were eliminated early in life in the primary lymphoid organs. This is achieved for T cells by negative selection in the thymus (see Fig. 10), and for some but not all B cells in the bone marrow.

Antigen presentation Any cells expressing MHC Class II are fully capable of binding self-peptides, but will only trigger T cells if they also express costimulatory molecules such as B7 (CD80/86) (see Fig. 14). Antigen presented in the absence of costimulation may trigger the T cell to receive a 'negative' signal and become unresponsive.

Immunological ignorance Some antigens (for example those in the chamber of the eye) do not normally induce self-reactivity simply because they never come into contact with cells of the normal immune system. This phenomenon is known as immunological ignorance. However, if the normal barriers are broken down, for example during a prolonged infection, these antigens can escape into the blood, and self-reactivity and damage of the tissue sometimes results.

B cell receptors (immunoglobulin) Exposure of B cells to high concentrations of antigen during their development leads either to clonal elimination (death of the B cell) or development of an unreactive 'anergic' B cell with little surface antibody. B cells against self antigens present at low concentrations (less than 10^{-5}M) survive, but are never normally activated because they require help from T cells to trigger antibody secretion. This mechanism also guards against mature B cells which subsequently change their specificity because of somatic mutation of their V genes (see Fig. 15), during an immune response. Thus B cell tolerance is determined by both 'central' tolerance (clonal deletion) and 'peripheral' tolerance (T cell regulated).

T cell receptors pass through an important selection process as they appear in the thymus, in which cells whose receptors have a sufficiently high affinity for self are clonally deleted. Some endogenous 'superantigens' such as mouse mammary tumour viruses can delete all T cells carrying a particular Vβ receptor chain. However, peripheral tolerance of T cells also occurs. The main mechanism for this is thought to be presentation of self antigens by cells which carry MHC but not the right costimulatory molecules. This can result in clonal elimination or sometimes 'anergy' in which the T cell simply becomes non-responsive.

Transgenic T or B cell receptor carrying mice Using transgenic technology, it has proved possible to create mice in which all B or T cells carry receptors of a single antigenic specificity. Despite the limitations of studying such artificial systems, these mice have been very important in demonstrating clearly clonal elimination and/or clonal anergy.

Suppressor cells T cells have been postulated to recognize and inhibit self-reactive lymphocytes, but the evidence is still controversial. However, there is no doubt that when self-reactivity has been artificially induced (see Fig. 36), T cells may develop to restore the status quo.

Induction of unreactivity towards non-self (tolerance)

Soluble antigen is less immunogenic and more 'tolerogenic', than antigen administered in the presence of adjuvants, because it does not activate antigen presenting cells to express the appropriate costimulatory molecules.

Fetal (or neonatal) administration of antigen was the first method shown to induce tolerance. It probably operates by a combination of clonal elimination and deficient antigen presentation, due perhaps to antigen presenting cell immaturity, but fetal B cells may also be particularly tolerizable because of differences in the way their Ig receptors are replaced (see above). There is some evidence that α fetoprotein, a major serum protein in the fetus, can inhibit self-reactive T cells.

Oral route Antigens absorbed through the gut are first 'seen' by liver macrophages, which remove immunogenic aggregates, etc., leaving only soluble 'tolerogen'. In addition, APC in the gut may be specialized for tolerance induction, to prevent immune responses against food. Trials are in progress to see whether administering self antigens (such as collagen for rheumatoid arthritis, or myelin basic protein for multiple sclerosis) can be used in the treatment of autoimmunity (see Fig. 36).

Antigen presenting cells APC are thought to exist in 'resting' and 'activated' states. Resting APC are thought to preferentially stimulate tolerance, while activation (e.g. by many microbial products, and cytokines produced during inflammation) favours immunogenicity.

Antibody induced tolerance Antibodies against some molecules on the surface of either T cells or APC can help to induce a state of tolerance. Tolerance induced in this is usually known as **enhancement**, from the ability to enhance the growth of tumours, transplants, etc. Antibodies to the CD4 molecule are particularly effective at inducing T cell tolerance to antigens given at the same time.

High doses of antigen are usually more tolerogenic, though repeated low doses can also induce tolerance in T cells. As a rule, T cell tolerance is easier to induce and lasts longer than B cell tolerance.

Antigen suicide Antigens coupled to toxic drugs, radioisotopes, etc., may home on to specific T or B cells and kill them without exposing other cells to danger. A similar principle has been tried to eliminate tumour cells using toxins coupled to antibodies (see Fig. 31).

Antigen–antibody complexes can sometimes induce tolerance by receptor blocking. However, complexes can also be highly immunogenic, depending on the exact nature and proportions of the antigen and the antibody.

Non-immunogenic carriers, such as 'self' material or non-degradeable molecules (e.g. D amino acids), can confer tolerogenicity on haptens that, on normal carriers, would be antigenic. This idea has been tried in allergy, to switch off specific IgE responses.

Anti-idiotype antibody has been tried in the treatment of autoimmunity and might be useful in transplantation. Unfortunately, however, suppressing one idiotype simply allows another antibody against the same antigen to take its place, so the usefulness of this approach is debatable (see Fig. 22).

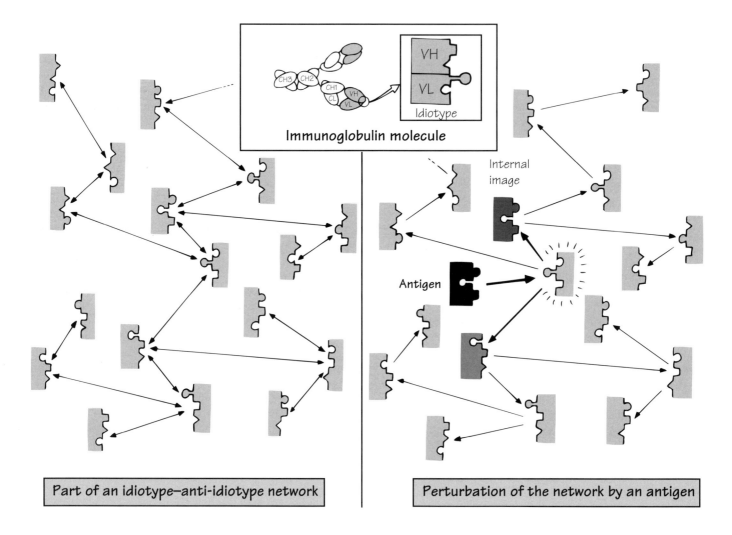

Part of an idiotype–anti-idiotype network

Perturbation of the network by an antigen

When we consider the enormous number of possible Ig and T cell receptor antigen-combining sites, designed to 'recognize' almost every conceivable molecular shape, it is hardly surprising that some of these receptors can recognize each other, and this can indeed be shown to happen. In such cases, we speak of one molecule as the **idiotype** and the other as the **anti-idiotype**; in theory either one could be an Ig or a TCR molecule. (The location of idiotypic determinants in the Ig molecule is shown stylistically at the top of the figure.)

This has several intriguing consequences. To begin with, it is clearly an example of self-reactivity or **autoimmunity**, which used to be thought impossible. Next, one might wonder what effect the anti-idiotype would have on the cell producing the idiotype, and vice versa, and thus on any immune response in which they are involved. Then again, it seems to challenge the old idea of 'antigens' and 'receptors' as two separate sets of molecules; now we can visualize, for example, an Ig receptor for a particular foreign antigen as being, at the same time, an antigen itself with respect to one or more other Ig molecules, which in turn are antigens for others . . . and so on. So that finally, if this chain is infinite, or virtually infinite, we arrive at the strange conclusion that

for every foreign antigen there must be a receptor molecule whose shape closely resembles it—the 'internal image'. In other words all *outside* shapes are also represented on the lymphocytes *inside* the body!

Looked at in this way, there is nothing really *foreign* about the antigens of bacteria, viruses, etc., and the interconnecting network of receptors can exist even in their absence (as shown in the left-hand figure). However, a foreign antigen, by inducing the formation of particular antibodies in increased amounts, will perturb this network (as shown in the right-hand figure), giving rise to a variety of idiotypes and anti-idiotypes, a few of which (darker shaded) may closely or partially resemble the original antigen.

The first person to spell out all these possibilities clearly was the great immunologist Neils Jerne, who in 1974 incorporated them into his Network Theory, whose ramifications have influenced immunology ever since. It is too early to say how many of the potential applications of this approach—in the regulation of immune responses, the treatment of autoimmunity and even the design of vaccines—will actually become established, but there are few immunological situations nowadays where network considerations do not enter into the discussion.

Evidence for the network

1 The injection of a single type of antibody (e.g. monoclonal) can induce the formation of anti-idiotypic antibodies (= anti-Ids) in the serum, detectable by their binding only to the inducing monoclonal (= Id).

2 Some anti-Ids will inhibit the binding between the Id and its inducing antigen, showing that they are directed against the actual antigen-binding site.

3 In an animal mounting an antibody response, the injection of anti-Id against one of the Ids of the response may inhibit further production of that Id (though not always, see 9 below).

4 During the later phases of an antibody response, particular anti-Ids may appear spontaneously at the time when the corresponding Ids decline.

Some problems

5 Experiments suggest that the network is not infinite, but probably consists of smaller sets of interconnecting Ids. It is possible that some B cells are connected via idiotype networks to self antigens, while others respond to non-self.

6 Some anti-Ids recognize Ids outside the antigen-binding site and do not inhibit antigen binding. Such Ids can also be found on other Ig molecules with a different specificity for antigen. Regulation by these anti-Ids would be Id-specific and not antigen-specific, and would not be of much value in controlling an actual immune response.

7 Furthermore, such Ids, induced by one antigen (e.g. a bacterial infection) might, via the network of Igs or of T helper cell receptors, lead to the formation of other Igs sharing the Id but with specificity for another antigen altogether. It has been suggested that this is one way in which autoantibodies may be induced (see Fig. 36)

8 The relationship between Ids and anti-Ids is rather similar to that between hormones and their receptors. Thus antibody to a hormone (e.g. insulin) may resemble the receptor and go on to induce antibodies to the receptor—a double dose of autoimmunity!

9 In experiments on regulation, injection of anti-Id sometimes inhibits and sometimes enhances the corresponding Id. The reason is not clear, but differences in Ig class or subclass and the details of the administration may all play a part.

Useful applications

10 If inhibition of Id production by injecting anti-Id could be made to work reproducibly, it might be a useful way of treating autoimmunity, allergy, etc., especially if it turns out that autoantibodies share particular Ids, as seems to be the case with some anti-DNA antibodies.

11 The most startling application of network theory, and possibly the most useful in the long run, concerns the **internal image** anti-Ids—those which resemble the inducing antigen (see figure). In certain cases, where the antigen is derived from an infectious organism and might be a useful vaccine, but is for some reason difficult to obtain in adequate amounts, it may be better to use the internal image anti-Id itself as a vaccine. This is a complex procedure involving the production of monoclonal Ids and then monoclonal anti-Ids, which have to be of the 'internal image' type, but it has given promising results, particularly with carbohydrate antigens—there being no need for the antigen and the anti-Id to have the same *structure* as long as they have a similar *shape*. A further advantage is that being proteins, these anti-Id vaccines might function as T-dependent antigens, inducing memory, etc., which carbohydrates typically do not.

23 **The cytokine network**

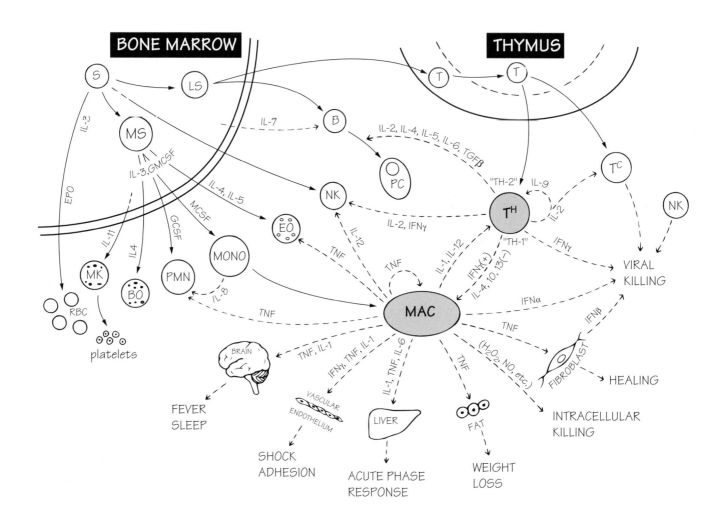

Frequent reference has been made in earlier sections to the small non-antigen-specific protein molecules that cells use to influence each other—for example the colony-stimulating factors (Fig. 4) and the interleukins (Figs 14, 18, 20)—and mention will be made in the sections on infection and tumours of other molecules of this general type such as interferon (Fig. 26) and tumour necrosis factor (TNF) (Fig. 31). Originally named lymphokines or monokines depending on the principal cell of origin, they are now collectively known as **cytokines**.

At one time it seemed that each of these molecules was designed for a particular purpose (viral inhibition, B cell differentiation, etc.) but now that most of them have been cloned and used in pure form, it is clear that they each have several different and apparently unrelated functions,

often overlapping and sometimes mutually synergistic or antagonistic, and can be responsible for harmful as well as beneficial effects during the course of various diseases.

The production and marketing of both cytokines and inhibitors of their action has therefore become a large and potentially lucrative business, and new ones are being discovered all the time. The figure has been simplified to show only more or less undisputed pathways. Production and activity are denoted by dashed lines, cell lineages by solid lines. To respond to a cytokine, a cell needs a specific surface **receptor**, and some of these have also been identified and cloned; possibly they will be useful as competitive inhibitors of cytokine action.

Interleukins

IL-1 (MW 17500) Formerly known as lymphocyte activating factor or endogenous pyrogen, IL-1 is a key regulator of inflammation, controlling body temperature, endothelial adhesion and macrophage activation. It shares many of its functions with TNF. There are two activating forms α and β, as well as an inhibitory analogue IL-1ra which acts as a competitive antagonist.

IL-2 (MW 15500) Originally designated T cell growth factor, IL-2 can stimulate many types of cell, including the ones making it, via a two-chain receptor.

IL-3 (MW 15000) or multi-CSF, stimulates the growth of the precursors of most types of marrow-derived cell, probably as an additional regulating element, and should really be classified as a Colony Stimulating Factor.

IL-4 (MW 20000) originally B cell growth factor 1, one of the T-helper factors for the antibody response characteristic of the T^{H2} subset, and essential for IgE production.

IL-5 (MW 45000) another T^{H2} cell derived B cell growth factor which also stimulates the maturation of eosinophils.

IL-6 (MW 26000) or B cell differentiation factor required for antibody secretion, is also an important mediator of the acute-phase inflammatory response.

IL-7 (MW 25000) is made by stromal marrow and thymus cells and stimulates early B and T cell growth.

IL-8 (MW 8500) its early name 'macrophage-derived neutrophil chemotactic factor' describes it admirably. Further molecules of this type have recently joined the IL family, see Chemokines, below.

IL-9 (MW 40000) A T cell-derived T cell growth factor

IL-10 (MW 40000) A T^{H2} cell product, generally inhibitory to cell-mediated responses.

IL-11 (MW 23000) Made in the bone marrow, with effects on stem cells, platelet production, and many inflammatory responses.

IL-12 (MW 70000) Produced predominantly by dendritic cells and macrophages, in response to microbial stimulation, it plays a key role in stimulating a T^{H1} response.

IL-13 (MW 12000) Like IL-4, a T^{H2} cell product that can inhibit macrophage responses.

IL-14 (MW 60000) A B cell growth factor produced by both B and T cells.

IL-15 (MW 11000) Like IL-2, predominantly a T cell growth factor.

IL-16 (MW 13000) Chemoattractant for T cells, eosinophils and monocytes.

IL-17 (MW 20000) Induces cytokine production by epithelia, endothelia and fibroblasts.

IL-18 (MW 23000) Like IL-12, induces IFN-γ and other T^{H1} like functions.

Interferons

IFNα (MW 20000) originally 'leucocyte-derived' IFN, a major inducer of antiviral proteins. It exists in over 20 closely similar subtypes.

IFNβ (MW 20000) originally 'fibroblast-derived' IFN. Like IFNα it is acid resistant and the two molecules share the same receptor.

IFNγ (MW 45000, normally dimerized) a quite different molecule from α and β, produced by lymphocytes and with a wide range of activities. It has been called Type II, acid-sensitive or 'immune' interferon. It is the major macrophage activator and considered to be characteristic of the T^{H1} subset. IFNs are more species-specific than most other cytokines.

Colony-stimulating factors

GM-CSF (MW 18–24000) is made by a variety of cells and stimulates granulocyte–macrophage precursors to increase both proliferative rate and function.

G-CSF (MW 19–22000) continues the maturation of granulocytes and has been found useful in raising neutrophil counts in patients (e.g. after irradiation).

M-CSF (MW 40–90000; often polymeric) preferentially stimulates monocyte and macrophage development and activity.

EPO (MW 36000) behaves like a cytokine in regulating red cell output, though unlike other cytokines it is made for this purpose only, and in a single location (the kidneys).

Tumour necrosis factors

TNFα (MW 17000; normally a trimer) Named for its ability to shrink some tumours by attacking their blood supply, TNF has widespread effects in inflammation, healing and—when produced in excess—vascular shock.

TNFβ (MW as TNFα) often known as lymphotoxin, it differs mainly in being mainly a lymphocyte product. Otherwise TNFα and β share a pair of receptors, considerable structure, and a chromosomal location within the MHC (see Fig. 13).

Chemokines

A very large family of small polypeptides, with names like MIP, MCP, MCAF, NAP, GRO, etc., which play a key role in chemotaxis and the regulation of leucocyte traffic (e.g. attracting neutrophils, lymphocytes and monocytes to inflammatory sites). There are three main classes of chemokines (α, β and γ) based on the distribution of conserved disulphide bonds. They bind to an equally large family of chemokine receptors, and the biology of the system is further complicated by the fact that many of the chemokines have multiple functions, and can bind to many different receptors.

Other cytokines not shown in figure

The definition of a cytokine is rather elastic, and shades over into classical hormones and various general growth and inhibitory factors, of which a few are of special interest to immunologists.

TGFβ (MW 25000) Transforming growth factors induce non-adherent growth in fibroblasts, but TGFβ has the additional property of inhibiting the activities of several cytokines, notably IL-2 and TNF. It may also be important in regulating IgA secretion by mucosal B cells.

Epidermal growth factor, nerve growth factor, and platelet-derived growth factor have a range of effects on repair and moulding of skin, bone, etc.

24 Immunity, hormones and the brain

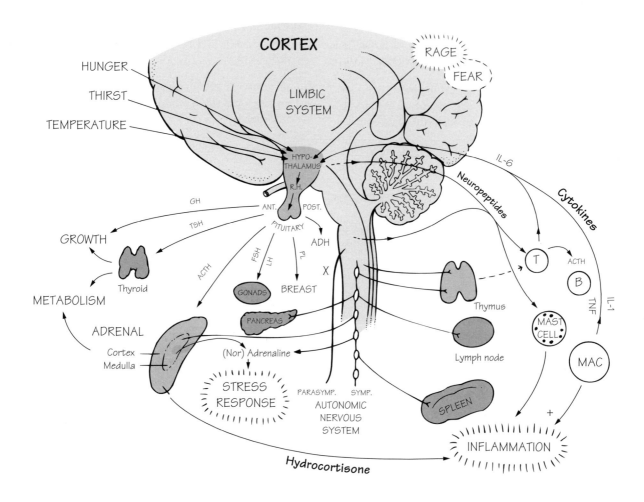

The language of immunology, with its emphasis on memory, tolerance, self and non-self, is reminiscent of that of neurology; indeed the immune system has been referred to as a 'mobile brain'. At the same time, the use of soluble 'messenger' molecules (see Fig. 23) by immune cells recalls the hormone-based organization of the endocrine system which is itself linked to the brain via the hypothalamic-pituitary-adrenal axis. Thus it has been suggested that all three systems can be seen as part of a single integrated network, known to its devotees by the cumbersome title of the psychoneuroimmunological, or neuroendocrino-immunological, system.

Evidence to support this comes from several directions. Stress, bereavement, etc., are known to lower lymphocyte responsiveness, and the same can be achieved by hypnosis and, some claim, by Pavlovian conditioning. Lymphoid organs receive a nerve supply from both sympathetic and parasympathetic systems, and the embryonic thymus is partly formed from brain, with which it shares antigens such as theta. Lymphocytes secrete several molecules normally thought of as either hormones or neuropeptides (see bottom right), while the effect of cytokines on the brain is well established (see Fig. 23).

At present, immunological opinion as to the significance of all this is divided. At one extreme are those who dismiss the connections as weak, trivial and irrelevant. At the other are the prophets of a new era of 'whole body' immunology stretching from the conscious mind to the antibody molecule–which would have significant implications for medical care. A middle-of-the-road view would be that such effects are the fine-tuning in a system that for the most part regulates itself autonomously. Time will tell who is nearest the truth.

Central nervous system

Cortex The outer layer of the brain in which conscious sensations, language, thought, and memory are controlled.

Limbic system An intermediate zone responsible for the more emotional aspects of behaviour.

Hypothalamus The innermost part of the limbic system, which regulates not only behaviour and mood but also vital physical functions such as food and water intake and temperature. It has connections to and from the cortex, brain stem, and endocrine system.

Pituitary gland The 'conductor of the endocrine orchestra', a gland about the size of a pea, divided into anterior and posterior portions secreting different hormones (see below).

RH Specific releasing hormones produced in the hypothalamus stimulate the pituitary to release its own hormones (e.g. TRH, TSH-releasing hormone).

Neuropeptides Small molecules responsible for some of the transmission of signals in the CNS. The hypothalamus produces several that cause pain (e.g. substance P) or suppress it (e.g. endorphins, encephalins).

Autonomic nervous system

In general, **sympathetic** nerves, via the secretion of noradrenaline (epinephrine), excite functions involved in urgent action ('fight or flight') such as cardiac output, respiration, blood sugar, awareness, sweating.

Parasympathetic nerves, many of which travel via cranial nerve **X** (the vagus), secrete acetylcholine and promote more peaceful activities such as digestion and close vision. Most viscera are regulated by one or the other or both. Massive sympathetic activation (including the adrenal medulla, see below), is triggered by fear, rage, etc.—the 'alarm' reaction which if allowed to become chronic, shades over into **stress**.

Endocrine system

Adrenal medulla The inner part of the adrenal gland, which when stimulated by sympathetic nerves releases **adrenaline**, with effects similar to noradrenaline but more prolonged.

Adrenal cortex The outer part of the adrenal gland, stimulated by corticotrophin (ACTH) from the anterior pituitary to secrete aldosterone, hydrocortisone (cortisol) and other hormones that regulate salt/water balance and protein and carbohydrate metabolism. In addition, hydrocortisone and its synthetic derivatives have powerful anti-inflammatory effects.

Thyroid Stimulated by thyrotrophin (TSH) from the anterior pituitary to release the iodine-containing thyroid hormones T3 and T4 (thyroxine) which regulate many aspects of cellular metabolism.

Growth hormone (GH) regulates the size of bones and soft tissues.

Gonads Two anterior pituitary hormones, follicle-stimulating (FSH) and luteinizing (LH) regulate the development of testes and ovaries, puberty, and the release of sex hormones. These changes are especially subject to hypothalamic influence—e.g. psychic, or, in animals, seasonal.

Posterior pituitary Here the main product is antidiuretic hormone (ADH), which retains water via the kidneys in response to osmotic receptors in the hypothalamus.

The **pancreas** and **parathyroids** function more or less autonomously to regulate glucose and calcium levels, respectively, although the pancreas also responds to autonomic nervous signals.

Immune system

(*Note:* the elements shown in the figure are all considered in detail elsewhere in this book. Here, attention is drawn only to the features linking them to the nervous and endocrine systems.)

Cytokines The most convincing immune–nervous system link is the induction of fever by TNF, IL-1, IFNs; high doses of many cytokines also cause drowsiness and general malaise. Cytokines, especially IL-2 and IL-6, are found in the brain. TNF and IL-1 are thought to induce ACTH secretion from the pituitary, probably via the hypothalamus.

Lymphoid organs Neurones terminating in the thymus and lymph nodes can be traced via sympathetic nerves to the spinal cord.

Lymphocytes have been shown to bear receptors for endorphins, encephalins and substance P, and also to secrete endorphins and hormones such as ACTH.

Immune responses are inhibited by hydrocortisone and sex hormones, and under stressful conditions, particularly when stress is inescapable, as with bereavement, examinations, etc. Hypnosis has been shown to inhibit immediate and delayed skin reactions. Whether corticosteroids can explain all such cases is a hotly debated point.

Autoimmunity It is remarkable how many autoimmune diseases (see Fig. 36) affect endocrine organs. Especially striking is the thyroid, where autoantibodies can both mimic and block the stimulating effect of TSH.

25 Anti-microbial immunity: a general scheme

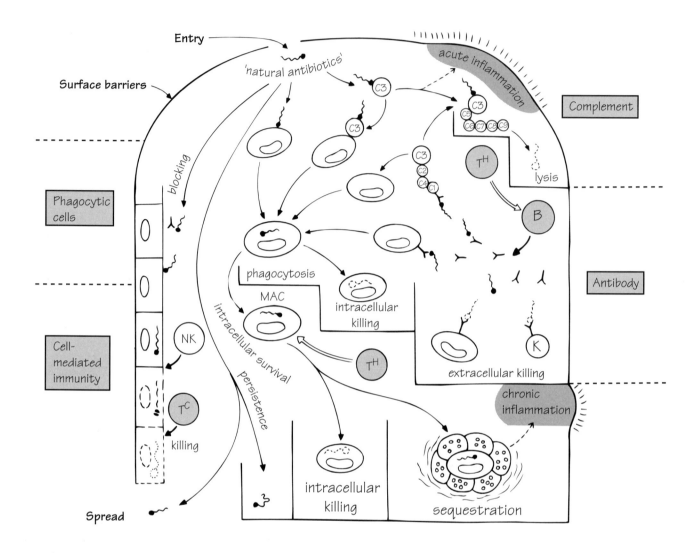

At this point the reader will appreciate that the immune system is highly efficient at recognizing **foreign** substances by their shape but has no infallible way of distinguishing whether or not they are **dangerous**. By and large, this approach works well to control infection, but it does have its unfortunate side—for example the violent immune response against foreign but harmless structures such as pollen grains, etc. (see Fig. 33).

Would-be parasitic micro-organisms that penetrate the barriers of skin or mucous membranes (top) have to run the gauntlet of four main recognition systems: **complement** (top right), **phagocytic cells** (centre), **antibody** (right), and **cell-mediated immunity** (bottom) together with their often interacting effector mechanisms. Unless primed by previous contact with the appropriate antigen, antibody and cell-mediated responses do not come into action for several days, whereas complement and phagocytic cells, being ever-present, act within minutes. There are also (top centre) specialized **natural** elements, such as lysozyme, interferon, etc., which act more or less non-specifically, much as **antibiotics** do.

Generally speaking, complement and antibody are most active against micro-organisms free in the blood or tissues, whilst cell-mediated responses are most active against those that seek refuge in cells (left). But which mechanism, if any, is actually effective, depends largely on the tactics of the micro-organism itself. Successful parasites are those able to evade, resist, or inhibit the relevant immune mechanisms, as illustrated in the following five figures.

Entry Many micro-organisms enter the body through wounds or bites, but others live on the skin or mucous membranes of the intestine, respiratory tract, etc., and are thus technically outside the body.

Surface barriers Skin and mucous membranes are to some extent protected by acid pH, enzymes, mucus, and other antimicrobial secretions, as well as IgA antibody (see below).

Natural antibiotics The antibacterial enzyme **lysozyme** (produced largely by macrophages, see Fig. 27) and the antiviral **interferons** (see Figs 23, 26) are responsible for a good deal of 'natural immunity' to what would otherwise be pathogenic organisms. Recent work has also identified another family of polypeptides with broad antimicrobial properties, produced especially at mucosal surfaces, and named **defensins**. This family of molecules is also found in many invertebrates (e.g. insects) and seems to represent an ancient component of innate immunity.

C3 Complement is activated directly ('alternative pathway') by many micro-organisms, leading to their lysis or phagocytosis. The same effect can also be achieved when C3 is activated by antibody ('classical pathway'; see Fig. 5) or by mannose-binding protein.

T^H Helper T cells perform several distinct functions in the immune response to microbes. Some respond to 'carrier' determinants and stimulate antibody synthesis by B cells. Viruses, bacteria, protozoa and worms have all been shown to function as fairly strong carriers, though there are a few organisms to which the antibody response appears to be T-independent. Others regulate 'delayed hypersensitivity' by secreting cytokines which attract and activate monocytes, eosinophils, etc. (see Figs 20, 23). The central role of T helper cells in almost all infections is shown by the serious effects of their destruction, e.g. in AIDS (see Fig. 40).

B Antibody formation by B lymphocytes is an almost universal feature of infection, of great diagnostic as well as protective value. As a general rule, IgM antibodies come first, then IgG and the other classes; IgM is therefore often a sign of recent infection. At mucous surfaces, IgA is the most effective antibody (see Fig. 16).

Blocking Where micro-organisms or their toxins need to enter cells, antibody may block this by combining with their specific attachment site. Tetanus and most viruses are examples. IgA in the intestine acts mainly in this way.

Phagocytosis by polymorphonuclear leucocytes or macrophages is the ultimate fate of most unsuccessful organisms. Both C3 and antibody tremendously improve this by attaching the microbe to the phagocytic cell through C3 or Fc receptors on the latter; this is known as 'opsonization' (see Fig. 8).

Intracellular killing Once inside the phagocytic cell, most organisms are killed and degraded by lysosomal enzymes. In certain cases, 'activation' of macrophages by T cells may be needed to trigger the killing process (see Fig. 20).

Extracellular killing Monocytes, polymorphs, and other killer (K) cells can kill antibody-coated cells *in vitro*, without phagocytosis; however, it is not clear how much this actually happens *in vivo*.

NK Natural killer cells are able to kill many virus-infected cells rapidly, but without the specificity characteristic of lymphocytes.

Intracellular survival Several important viruses, bacteria and protozoa can survive inside macrophages, where they resist killing. Other organisms survive within cells of muscle, liver, brain, etc. In such cases, antibody cannot attack them and cell-mediated responses are the only hope.

T^C Cytotoxic T cell, specialized for killing, by lysis, 'self' cells altered by viruses, etc., and also allogeneic (e.g. grafted) cells (see Fig. 20), and perhaps tumours (Fig. 31).

Sequestration Micro-organisms which cannot be killed (e.g. some mycobacteria) or products which cannot be degraded (e.g. streptococcal cell walls) can be walled off by the formation of a granuloma by macrophages, often aided by cell-mediated immune responses (see Fig. 20).

Spread Successful micro-organisms must be able to leave the body and infect another one. Coughs and sneezes, faeces and insect bites are the commonest modes of spread.

Persistence Some very successful parasites are able to escape all the above-mentioned immunological destruction mechanisms by sophisticated protective devices of their own. Needless to say, these constitute some of the most chronic and intractable infectious diseases.

Inflammation Although some micro-organisms cause tissue damage directly (e.g. cytopathic viruses or the toxins of staphylococci), it is unfortunately true that much of the tissue damage resulting from infection is due to the response of the host. Acute and chronic inflammation are discussed in detail elsewhere (Figs 6, 35), but it is worth noting here that infectious organisms frequently place the host in a real dilemma: whether to eliminate the infection at all costs or to limit tissue damage and allow some of the organisms to survive. Given enough time, natural selection should arrive at the balance which is best for both parasite and host.

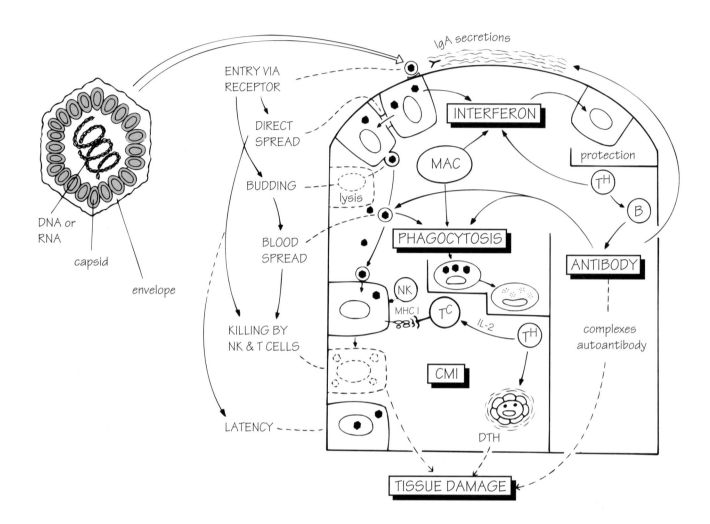

Viruses differ from all other infectious organisms in being much smaller (see Fig. 42) and lacking cell walls and independent metabolic activity, so that they are unable to replicate outside the cells of their host. The key process in virus infection is therefore **intracellular replication**, which may or may not lead to cell death. In the figure, viruses are depicted as hexagons, but in fact their size and shape are extremely varied.

For rapid protection, **interferon** (top) plays the same 'natural antibiotic' role as lysozyme in bacterial infection, though the mechanism is quite different. Antibody (right) is valuable in preventing entry and blood-borne spread of some viruses, but the ability of others to spread from cell to cell (left) puts the burden of adaptive immunity on the cytotoxic T cell system, which specializes in recognizing altered 'self' MHC Class I antigens and the NK cells, which seem to kill best when there is little or no MHC on the infected cell, and come into action more rapidly than T^C cells. Macrophages play a variety of roles: by secreting interferon, or by phagocytosis. The antibody-forming system can also respond to altered self, often producing antiself (auto-) antibodies in the process (see Fig. 36).

Note that tissue damage may result from either the virus itself or the host immune response to it. In the long run, no parasite that seriously damages or kills its host can count on its own survival, so that adaptation, which can be very rapid in viruses, generally tends to be in the direction of decreased virulence. But infections that are well adapted to their normal animal host can occasionally be highly virulent to humans; rabies (dogs), and Marburg virus (monkeys) are examples of this ('zoonosis').

Intermediate between viruses and bacteria are those obligatory intracellular organisms which do possess cell walls (*Rickettsia*, *Trachoma*) and others without walls but capable of extracellular replication (*Mycoplasma*). Immunologically, the former are closer to viruses, the latter to bacteria.

Receptors All viruses need to interact with specific receptors on the cell surface; examples where the receptor has been identified include Epstein–Barr virus (EBV) (CR2 on cells), rabies (acetylcholine receptor on neurones) and measles (CD46 on cells).

Interferon A group of proteins (see Fig. 23) produced in response to virus infection (and also bacterial **LPS**, etc.) which stimulates cells to make proteins that block viral transcription, and thus protects them from infection.

T^C, NK, CMI As described in Figs 13, 17 and 20, cytotoxic T cells 'learn' to recognize Class I MHC antigens, and then respond to these in association with virus antigens on the cell surface. It was during the study of antiviral immunity in mice that the central role of the MHC in T cell responses was discovered. NK cells can destroy some virus-infected cells, but are not MHC restricted. The role of DTH in viral infection, via macrophage activation, remains controversial.

Antibody Specific antibody can bind to virus and thus block its ability to bind to its specific receptor and hence infect cells. This is called neutralization. Neutralizing antibody is probably an important part of protection against many viruses, including such common infections as influenza.

Viruses

There is no proper taxonomy for viruses, which can be classified according to: size, shape, the nature of their genome (DNA or RNA), how they spread (budding, cytolysis or directly; all are illustrated), and—of special interest here—whether they are eliminated or merely driven into hiding by the immune response. Brief details of some important viruses are given below.

Pox viruses (smallpox, vaccinia) Large; DNA; spread locally, avoiding antibody, as well as in blood leucocytes; express antigens on the infected cell, attracting CMI. The antigenic cross-reaction between these two viruses is the basis for the use of vaccinia to protect against smallpox (Jenner, 1798, but known in the Far East for thousands of years). Thanks to this vaccine, smallpox is the first disease ever to have been eliminated from the entire globe. Severe T cell deficiency (see Fig. 39) often presents as a progressive fatal inability to control vaccinia.

Herpes viruses (herpes simplex, varicella, EBV, CMV (cytomegalovirus)) Medium; DNA; tend to persist and cause different symptoms when reactivated: thus varicella (chicken-pox) reappears as zoster (shingles); EB (infectious mononucleosis) may initiate malignancy (Burkitt's lymphoma; see Fig. 31) CMV has become important as an opportunist infection in immunosuppressed patients.

Adenoviruses (throat and eye infections) Medium; DNA. Numerous antigenically different types make immunity very inefficient and vaccination a problem.

Myxoviruses (influenza, mumps, measles) Large; RNA; spread by budding. Influenza is the classic example of attachment by specific receptor (haemagglutinin) and also of antigenic variation, which accounts for the relative uselessness of adaptive immunity. Mumps, by spreading in the testis, can initiate autoimmune damage. Measles infects lymphocytes, causes non-specific suppression of CMI, and persists to cause

SSPE (subacute sclerosing panencephalitis); some feel that multiple sclerosis may also be a disease of this type.

Rubella ('German measles') Medium; RNA. A mild disease feared for its ability to damage the fetus in the first 4 months of pregnancy. An attenuated vaccine gives good immunity.

Rabies Large; RNA. Spreads via nerves to the central nervous system, usually following a dog bite. Passive antibody can be life-saving.

Arboviruses (yellow fever) Arthropod-borne; small; RNA. Blood spread to the liver leads to jaundice. Good immunity and protection by vaccine.

Enteroviruses (polio) Small; RNA. Only 'seen' by the immune system on entry (via the gut) and when the host cell is lysed, and therefore susceptible to antibody (including IgA) but not CMI.

Rhinoviruses (common cold) Small; RNA. As with adenoviruses there are too many serotypes for antibody-mediated immunity to be effective.

Hepatitis can be caused by at least six viruses, including A (infective; RNA), B (serum-transmitted; DNA) and C (previously known as 'non-A non-B; RNA). In hepatitis B, immune complexes and autoantibodies are found, and virus can persist in 'carriers', particularly in tropical countries, where it is strongly associated with cirrhosis and cancer of the liver. Prolonged treatment with IFNα may ameliorate the carrier state. However, very effective vaccines are now available for uninfected adults, both for Hepatitis A and B.

Arenaviruses (Lassa fever) Medium; RNA. A disease of rats often fatal in man. A somewhat similar zoonosis is Marburg disease of monkeys.

Retroviruses (tumours) RNA. Contain reverse transcriptase, which allows insertion into the infected cell's DNA. The human T cell leukaemia viruses (HTLV) and the AIDS virus HIV belong to this group (see Fig. 40).

Trachoma An organism of the psittacosis group (*Chlamydia*). The frightful scarring of the conjunctiva may be due to over-vigorous CMI.

Typhus and other *Rickettsia* may survive in macrophages, like the tubercle bacillus.

Prions These are, strictly speaking, not viruses at all, but host proteins, which under certain circumstances can be induced to polymerize spontaneously to form small virus-like particles called 'prions'. These prions are found predominantly in the brain, and can cause progressive brain-damage (hence their original classification as 'slow viruses'). The first example of a 'prion' disease was **Kuru**, a progressive brain disease spread only by cannibalism. However, prion diseases are now thought to be responsible for scrapie, and most notoriously for the UK epidemic of bovine spongiform encephalopathy (BSE or 'mad cow disease') and the human equivalent Creutzfeld-Jacob disease (CJD). Many aspects of prion disease remain poorly understood and there is no known treatment. There appears to be little or no immune response to prions, perhaps because they are 'self' molecules.

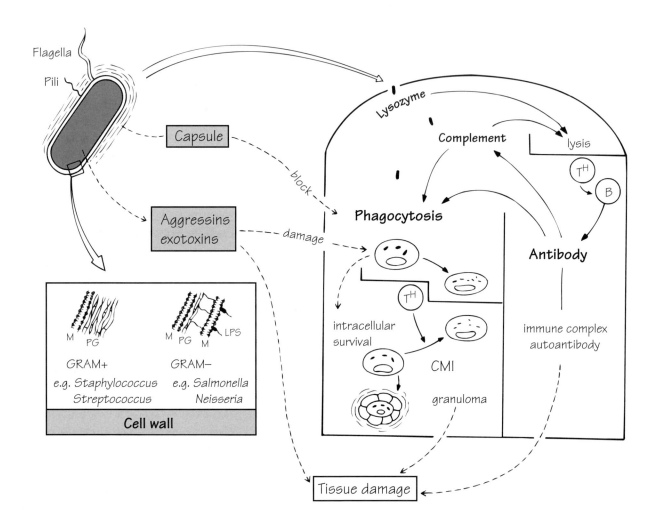

Unlike viruses, bacteria are cellular organisms, mostly capable of fully independent life, though some have unfortunately chosen to be parasitic on larger animals some or all of the time. Together with viruses, they constitute the major infectious threat to health in developed countries. Since the discovery of the antibiotics in the 1930s and 1940s bacterial infection has been controlled largely by chemotherapy. However, with the recent rise in antibiotic-resistant strains of bacteria, there is renewed interest in developing new or improved vaccines against the bacteria responsible for such diseases as tuberculosis, meningitis and food-poisoning.

The usual destiny of unsuccessful bacteria is death by **phagocytosis**; survival therefore entails avoidance of this fate. The main ways in which a bacterium (top left) can achieve this lie in the **capsule** (affecting attachment), the **cell wall** (affecting digestion) and the release of **exotoxins** (which damage phagocytic and other cells). Fortunately most capsules and toxins are strongly antigenic and antibody overcomes many of their effects; this is the basis of the majority of anti-

bacterial vaccines. In the figure, processes beneficial to the bacteria or harmful to the host are shown in broken lines.

Bacteria are prokaryocytes, unlike higher organisms from fungi to man (which are eukaryocytes) and this means that their structures and molecules are more foreign to us than fungi, protozoa, and worms; thus there is more chance of our evolving defences that attack the parasite and not the host. On the host side, the 'natural antibiotic' **lysozyme** represents perhaps the furthest point achieved in elaborating substances that attack bacteria but not host cells (until the antibiotic era; it is interesting that both lysozyme and penicillin were discovered by Sir Alexander Fleming).

As with viruses, some of the most virulent and obstinate bacterial infections are zoonoses—plague (rats) and brucellosis (cattle) being examples. Bacteria that manage to survive in macrophages (e.g. TB) can induce severe immune-mediated tissue damage (see Fig. 35); indeed the delayed hypersensitivity skin reaction characteristic of T cell immunity in general was for many years referred to as 'bacterial allergy'.

Cell wall   Outside their plasma membrane (M in the figure) bacteria have a cell wall composed of a mucopeptide called peptidoglycan (PG); it is here that lysozyme acts by attacking the *N*-acetyl muramic acid–*N*-acetyl glucosamine links. In addition, Gram-negative bacteria have a second membrane with lipopolysaccharides (LPS, also called endotoxin) inserted in it.

Flagella, the main agent of bacterial motility, contain highly antigenic proteins (the 'H antigens' of typhoid, etc.) which give rise to immobilizing antibody.

Pili are used by bacteria to adhere to cells; antibody can prevent this (e.g. IgA against gonococcus).

Capsule   Many bacteria owe their virulence to capsules, which protect them from contact with phagocytes. Most are large branched polysaccharide molecules, but some are protein. It is interesting that many of these capsular polysaccharides, and also some proteins from flagella, are T-independent antigens (see Fig. 17). Since T-independent antibody is thought to have preceded the T-dependent type in evolution (see Fig. 3), this fits in with the idea that bacteria were the main driving force for the development of the antibody-forming system. Examples of capsulated bacteria are pneumococcus, meningococcus and *Haemophilus*.

Exotoxins   (as distinct from the **endotoxin** (LPS) of cell walls). Gram-positive bacteria often secrete proteins with destructive effects on phagocytes, local tissues, the CNS, etc.; frequently these are the cause of death. In addition there are proteins collectively known as **aggressins** which help the bacteria to spread by dissolving host tissue.

Sepsis   Occasionally, uncontrolled systemic responses to bacterial infection develop, which can lead to rapid life-threatening disease. Such responses are still an important cause of death after major surgery. Overproduction of TNF-α, especially by macrophages, plays a major role in these reactions.

Bacteria

In the figure, bacteria are given their popular rather than their proper taxonomic names. Some individual aspects of interest are listed below:

Strep.   *Streptococcus*, classified either by haemolytic exotoxins (α, β, γ) or cell wall antigens (groups A–Q). Group A, β-haemolytic are the most pathogenic, possessing capsules (M protein) that attach to mucous membranes but resist phagocytosis, numerous exotoxins (whence scarlet fever), indigestible cell walls causing severe cell-mediated reactions, antigens that cross-react with cardiac muscle (rheumatic fever), and a tendency to kidney-damaging immune complexes.

Staph.   *Staphylococcus*. Antiphagocytic factors include the fibrin-forming enzyme coagulase and protein A, which binds to the Fc portion of IgG, blocking opsonization. Numerous other toxins make staphylococci highly destructive, abscess-forming organisms.

Pneumococcus, meningococcus   Typed by the polysaccharides of their capsules, and especially virulent in the tropics, where vaccines made from their capsular polysaccharides are proving highly effective in preventing epidemics. Patients with deficient antibody responses (see Fig. 39) are particularly prone to these infections.

Gonococcus   IgA may block attachment to mucous surfaces, but the bacteria secrete a protease which destroys the IgA; thus the infection is seldom eliminated, leading to a 'carrier' state. Bacteria of this type are the only ones definitely shown to be disposed of by complement-mediated lysis.

Mycobacterium tuberculosis; leprosy   These mycobacteria have very tough cell walls, rich in lipids, which resist intracellular killing; they can also inhibit phagosome–lysosome fusion. Chronic CMI results, with tissue destruction and scarring. In leprosy, a 'spectrum' between localization and dissemination corresponds to a predominance of CMI and of antibody, respectively.

Shigella and **cholera** are confined to the intestine, and produce their effects by secreting exotoxins. However, antitoxin vaccines are much less effective than natural infection in inducing immunity, and attempts are being made to produce strains attenuated by genetic manipulations (see Fig. 41).

Salmonella (e.g. **S. typhi**) infects the intestine but can also survive and spread within macrophages.

Tetanus owes its severity to the rapid action of its exotoxin on the CNS. Antibody ('antitoxin') is highly effective at blocking toxin action—an example where neither complement nor phagocytic cells are needed.

Diphtheria also secretes powerful neurotoxins, but death can be due to local tissue damage in the larynx ('false membrane').

Syphilis should be mentioned as an example of bacteria surviving all forms of immune attack without sheltering inside cells. Autoantibody to mitochondrial cardiolipin is the basis of the Wasserman reaction. Cross-reactions of this type, due presumably to bacterial attempts to mimic host antigens and thus escape the attentions of the immune system, are clearly a problem to the host, who has to choose between ignoring the infection and making autoantibodies which may be damaging to his own tissues; see Fig. 36 for further discussion of autoimmunity.

Borrelia, another spirochaete, has the property (found also with some viruses and protozoa) of varying its surface antigens to confuse the host's antibody-forming system. As a result, waves of infection are seen ('relapsing fever').

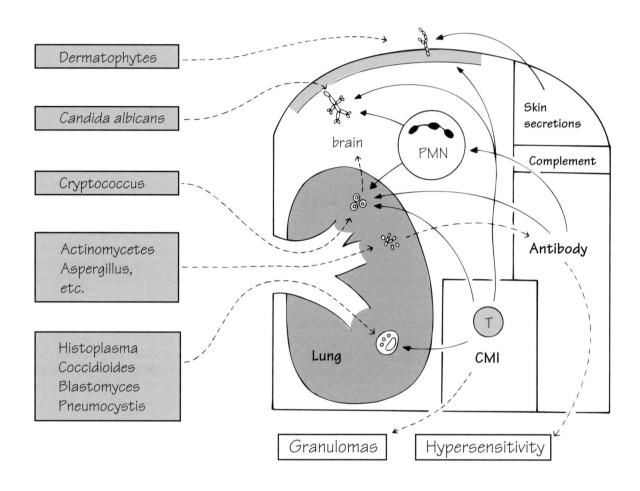

The vast majority of fungi are free-living, but a few can colonize larger animals, particularly if exposure is intense (e.g. farmers) or the immune system is in some way compromised (e.g. AIDS).

Fungal infections are normally only a superficial nuisance (e.g. ringworm: top), but a few fungi can cause serious systemic disease, usually entering via the lung in the form of spores (centre left); the outcome depends on the degree and type of immune response, and may range from an unnoticed respiratory episode to rapid fatal dissemination or a violent hypersensitivity reaction.

In general, the survival mechanisms of successful fungi are similar to those of bacteria: antiphagocytic capsules (e.g. *Cryptococcus*), resistance to digestion within macrophages (e.g. *Histoplasma*, etc.), and destruction of polymorphs (e.g. *Coccidioides*). Some yeasts activate complement via the alternative pathway, but it is not known if this has any effect on survival.

Perhaps the most interesting fungus from the immunological point of view is ***Candida albicans*** (upper left), a common and harmless inhabitant of skin and mucous membranes which readily takes advantage of any weakening of host resistance. This is most strikingly seen when polymorphs (PMN) or T cells are defective, but it also occurs in patients who are undernourished, immunosuppressed, iron deficient, alcoholic, diabetic, aged or simply 'run down' (see Fig. 39). Organisms that thrive only in the presence of immunodeficiency are called 'opportunists' and they include not only fungi but several viruses (e.g. CMV), bacteria (e.g. pseudomonas), protozoa (e.g. toxoplasma) and worms (e.g. strongyloides) and their existence testifies to the unobtrusive efficiency of the normal immune system.

PMN Polymorphonuclear leucocyte ('neutrophil'), an important phagocytic cell. Recurrent fungal as well as bacterial infections may be due to defects in PMN numbers or function, which may in turn be genetic or drug-induced (steroids, antibiotics). Functional defects may affect chemotaxis ('lazy leucocyte'), phagolysosome formation (Chediak–Higashi syndrome), peroxide production (chronic granulomatous disease), myeloperoxidase and other enzymes. Deficiencies in complement or antibody will of course also compromise phagocytosis (see also Fig. 39).

T Since severe fungal infection in both the skin and mucous membranes (*candida*) and in the lung (*pneumocystis*) are common in T cell deficiencies, T cells evidently have antifungal properties, but the precise mechanism is not clear. Some fungi (see below) can apparently also be destroyed by NK cells.

Hypersensitivity reactions are a feature of many fungal infections, especially those infecting the lung. They are mainly of Type I or IV (see Fig. 33 for an explanation of what this means).

Dermatophytes Filamentous fungi which metabolize keratin and therefore live off skin, hair and nails (ring-worm). Sebaceous secretions help to control them, but CMI may also play an ill-defined part.

Candida albicans (*Monilia*); a yeast-like fungus which causes severe spreading infections of the skin, mouth, etc. in patients with immunodeficiency, especially T cell defects. Remarkable clinical improvement, together with restoration of a positive delayed hypersensitivity skin test, has been induced by 'transfer factor', an extract of normal leucocytes originally believed to confer specific T cell responsiveness but now thought to be non-antigen-specific, albeit effective. The precise role of T cells in controlling this infection is not understood.

Cryptococcus h A capsulated yeast able to resist phagocytosis unless opsonized by antibody and/or complement (cf. *Pneumococcus*, etc.). In immunodeficient patients, spread to the brain and meninges is a serious complication. The organisms can be killed at least *in vitro*, by NK cells.

Actinomycetes and other sporing fungi from mouldy hay, etc. can reach the lung alveoli, stimulate antibody production and subsequently induce severe hypersensitivity ('farmer's lung'). Both IgG and IgE may be involved. **Aspergillus** is particularly prone to cause trouble in patients with tuberculosis.

Histoplasma (histoplasmosis), **Coccidioides** (coccidioidomycosis), and **Blastomyces** (blastomycosis) are similar in causing pulmonary disease, particularly in America, which may either heal spontaneously, disseminate body-wide, or progress to chronic granulomatosis and fibrosis, depending on the immunological status of the patient. The obvious resemblance to tuberculosis and leprosy emphasizes the point that it is microbial survival mechanisms (in this case, resistance to digestion in macrophages) rather than taxonomic relationships, which determine the pattern of disease.

Pneumocystis carinii is mentioned here because, though it was originally assumed to be a protozoan, studies of its RNA suggest that it is nearer to the fungi. Pneumocystis pneumonia has become one of the most feared complication of AIDS (see Fig. 40), which suggests that T cells normally prevent its proliferation, though the mechanism is unknown.

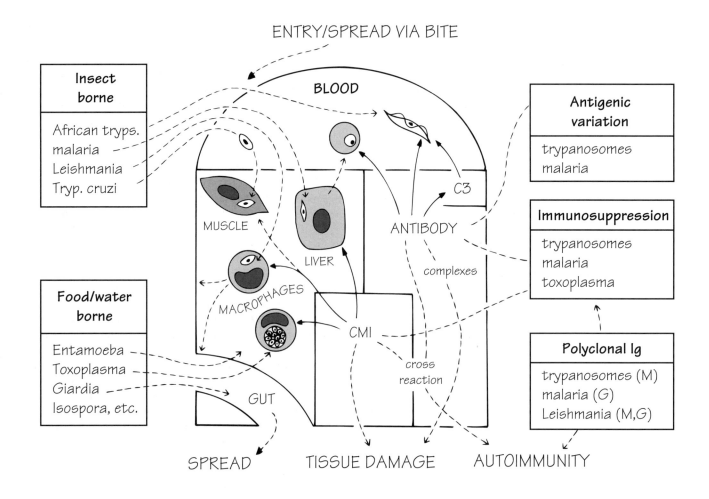

Relatively few (less than 20) protozoa infest man, but among these are four of the most formidable parasites of all, in terms of numbers affected and severity of disease: malaria, the African and American trypanosomes, and *Leishmania* (top left). These owe their success to combinations of strategy also found among bacteria and viruses — long-distance **spread** by insect vectors (cf. plague, typhus, yellow fever), **intracellular** habitat (shaded in figure; cf. tuberculosis, viruses), **antigenic variation** (cf. influenza) and **immunosuppression** (cf. HIV) but they are so highly developed that complete acquired resistance to protozoal infections is quite exceptional, and what immunity there is

often serves merely to keep parasite numbers down ('premunition') and the host alive, to the advantage of the parasite. The rationale for vaccination is correspondingly weak, especially since some of the symptoms of these diseases appear to be due to the immune response rather than to the parasite itself.

By contrast, the intestinal protozoa (bottom left) generally cause fairly mild disease, except when immunity is deficient or suppressed. Nevertheless, together with the intestinal worm infections described on the next page, they add up to a tremendous health burden on the inhabitants of tropical countries.

African trypanosomes *Trypanosoma gambiense* and *T. rhodesiense*, carried by tsetse flies, cause sleeping sickness in West and East Africa, respectively. The blood form, though susceptible to antibody and complement, survives by repeatedly replacing its surface coat of glycoprotein 'variant antigen' by a gene-switching mechanism; the number of variants is unknown but large (perhaps as many as 1000). High levels of non-specific IgM, including autoantibodies, coexist with suppressed antibody responses to other antigens such as vaccines; this may be due to polyclonal activation of B cells by a parasite product (cf. bacterial lipopolysaccharides). Humans are resistant to the trypanosomes of rodents because of a normal serum factor (high-density lipoprotein; HDL) which agglutinates them—a striking example of natural immunity.

Malaria *Plasmodium falciparum* (the most serious), *P. malariae*, *P. vivax* and *P. ovale* are transmitted by mosquitoes. There is a brief liver stage, against which some immunity can be induced, probably via cytotoxic T cells, followed by a cyclical invasion of red cells, against which antibody is partially effective; antigenic variation and polyclonal IgG production may account for the slow development of immunity. Vaccination protects against the red cell stage in certain animal models, and also against the sexual gamete state. There has been continued, but so far largely unsuccessful interest in the possibility of producing a vaccine against *P. falciparium* in man, although some moderately encouraging trials having been carried out. Human red cells lacking the Duffy blood group, or containing fetal haemoglobin, are 'naturally' resistant to *P. vivax* and *P. falciparum*, respectively. *P. malariae* is specially prone to induce immune complex deposition in the kidney. High levels of the cytokine TNF (see Fig. 23) are found in severe cases of malaria, and this may represent over-stimulation of macrophages by a parasite product—a form of pathology also seen in Gram-negative bacterial septicaemia (see Fig. 32). Malaria was one of the first diseases to be experimentally treated by the use of anti-TNF antibody.

Babesia or piroplasms, are tick-borne cattle parasites resembling malaria, which occasionally infect man, particularly following removal of the spleen or immunosuppressive therapy. In cattle and dogs an attenuated vaccine has been strikingly successful.

Theileria (East Coast fever) a cattle infection resembling malaria except that the 'liver' stage occurs in lymphocytes, is unusual in being killed by cytotoxic T cells—that is, behaving essentially like a virus.

Leishmania a confusing variety of parasites, carried by sandflies, which cause an even more bewildering array of diseases in different parts of the tropics. The organisms inhabit macrophages, and the pathology (mainly in the skin and viscera) seems to depend on the strength of cell-mediated immunity and/or its balance with antibody (cf. leprosy). Cutaneous leishmaniasis in Africa is unusual in stimulating self-cure and subsequent resistance. This example of protection has apparently been known and applied in the Middle East for many centuries ('leishmanization'). There is evidence from mouse experiments that resistance is mediated by T^{H1} cells and can be compromised by T^{H2} cells, and also that nitric oxide (see Fig. 8) may be a major killing element.

Trypanosoma cruzi, the cause of Chagas' disease in Central and South America, is transmitted from animal reservoirs by reduviid bugs. It infects many cells, notably cardiac muscle and autonomic nervous ganglia. There is some suggestion that cell-mediated autoimmunity against normal cardiac muscle may be responsible for the chronic heart failure, and similarly with the nervous system, where uptake of parasite antigens by neurones and actual similarity between host and parasite have both been shown to occur. The organism has been killed *in vitro* by antibody and eosinophils, but the only prospect for vaccination seems to be against the blood stage. A better prospect would be to get rid of the poor housing in which the vector flourishes.

Toxoplasma *T. gondii* is particularly virulent in the fetus and immunosuppressed patients, chiefly affecting the brain and eye. It can survive inside macrophages by preventing phagolysosome formation (cf. tuberculosis), but cell-mediated immunity can overcome this. *Toxoplasma* stimulates macrophages and suppresses T cells, leading to varied effects on resistance to other infections.

Entamoeba histolytica normally causes disease in the colon (amoebic dysentery), but can get via the blood to the liver, etc., and cause dangerous abscesses by direct lysis of host cells. Some animals, and perhaps man, may develop a degree of immunity to these tissue stages but not to the intestinal disease.

Giardia, Balantidium, Cryptosporidium, Isospora, etc. normally restrict their effects to the gut, causing dysentery and occasionally malabsorption, but can be a severe complication of AIDS (see Fig. 40).

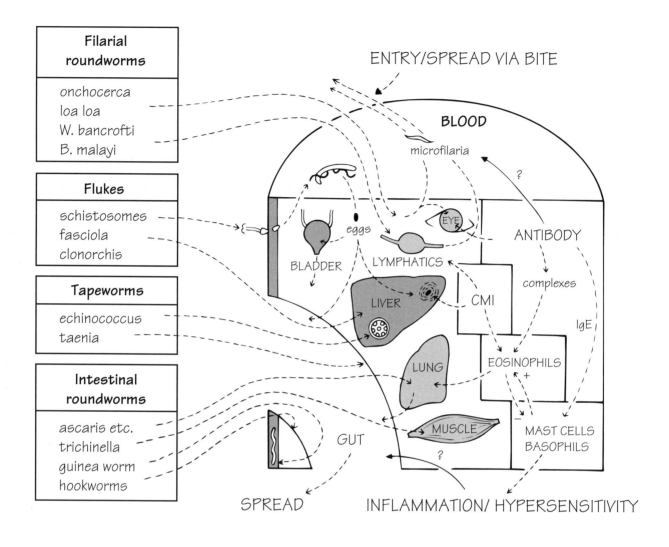

Parasitic worms of all three classes (roundworms, tapeworms and flukes) are responsible for numerous human diseases, including three of the most unpleasant (upper left): onchocerciasis, elephantiasis and schistosomiasis. These worms are transmitted with the aid of specific insect or snail vectors, and are restricted to the tropics, while the remainder (lower left) can be picked up anywhere by eating food contaminated with their eggs, larvae or cysts. A feature of many worm infections is their complex life cycles and circuitous migratory patterns, during which they often take up residence in a particular organ (shaded in figure).

Another striking feature is the predominance of **eosinophils** and of **IgE**; as a result, hypersensitivity reactions in skin, lung, etc., are common, but whether they are ever protective is still controversial. Since they do not replicate in the human host (unlike protozoa, bacteria and viruses), individual worms must resist the immune response particularly well in order to survive, and, as with the best-adapted protozoa (cf. malaria), immunity operates, if at all, to keep down the numbers of worms rather than to eliminate them. The outlook for vaccination might seem very dim, but it is surprisingly effective in certain dog and cattle infections.

Mystifying, but provocative, is the finding that several drugs originally used against worms (niridazole, levamisole, hetrazan) turn out to have suppressive or stimulatory effects on T cells, inflammation, and other immunological elements, bringing out the point that worms are highly developed animals and share many structures and pathways with their hosts.

Eosinophils may have three effects in worm infections; phagocytosis of the copious antigen–antibody complexes, modulation of hypersensitivity by inactivation of mediators, and (*in vitro*, at least) killing of certain worms with the aid of IgG antibody. Eosinophilia is partly due to mast cell and T cell chemotactic factors; T cells may also stimulate output from the bone marrow via cytokines such as IL-5.

IgE Worms, and even some worm extracts, stimulate specific and non-specific IgE production; it has been suggested but not proved that the resulting inflammatory response (e.g. in the gut) may hinder worm attachment or entry. There is also a belief that the high IgE levels, by blocking mast cells, can prevent allergy to pollen, etc. Production of IgE is considered to reflect the activity of T^{H2} helper cells.

Roundworms (nematodes)

Nematodes may be filarial (in which the first-stage larva, or microfilaria, can only develop in an insect, and only the third stage is infective to man), or intestinal (in which full development can occur in the patient).

Filarial nematodes *Onchocerca volvulus* is spread by *Simulium* flies, which deposit larvae and collect microfilariae in the skin. Microfilaria also inhabit the eye, causing 'river blindness' which may be largely due to immune responses. In the Middle East, pathology is restricted to the skin; parasitologists and immunologists disagree as to whether this reflects different species or a disease spectrum (cf. leprosy). *Loa loa* (loasis) is somewhat similar but less severe. *Wuchereria bancrofti* and *Brugia malayi* are spread by mosquitoes, which suck microfilariae from the blood. The larvae inhabit lymphatics, causing elephantiasis, partly by blockage and partly by inducing cell-mediated immune responses; soil elements (e.g. silicates) may also be involved. In some animal models, microfilaraemia can be controlled by antibody.

Intestinal nematodes *Ascaris, Strongyloides, Toxocara.* Travelling through the lung, larvae may cause asthma, etc., associated with eosinophilia. *Trichinella spiralis* larvae encyst in muscles. In some animal models, worms of this type stimulate good protective immunity. *Strongyloides* has become an important cause of disease in immunosuppressed patients. *Toxocara*, picked up from dogs or cats, is an important cause of widespread disease in young children, and eye damage in older ones.

Guinea worms (*Dracunculus*) live under the skin and can be up to 4 feet long. **Hookworms** (*Ancylostoma, Necator*) enter through the skin and live in the small intestine on blood, causing severe anaemia. None of these worms appear to stimulate useful immunity.

Flukes (trematodes)

Trematodes spend part of their life cycle in a snail, from which the cercariae infect man either by penetrating the skin (**Schistosoma**) or by being eaten (**Fasciola, Clonorchis**). The latter ('liver flukes') inhabit the liver but do not induce protective immunity.

Schistosomes ('blood flukes') live and mate harmlessly in venous blood (*Schistosoma mansoni, S. japonicum*: mesenteric; *S. haematobium*: bladder), only causing trouble when their eggs are trapped in the liver or bladder, where strong granulomatous T cell-mediated reactions lead to fibrosis in the liver and nodules and sometimes cancer in the bladder. The adult worms evade immune attack by covering their surface with antigens derived from host cells, at the same time stimulating antibody which may destroy subsequent infections at an early stage. Eosinophils, macrophages, IgG and IgE have all been implicated. Schistosomes also secrete a variety of molecules which destroy host antibodies and inhibit macrophages, etc., making the adult worm virtually indestructible. The combination of adult survival with killing of young forms is referred to as 'concomitant immunity'.

Fasciola are chiefly a problem in farm animals, where they live in the bile duct. What immunity there is appears to lead mainly to liver damage and vaccines have been disappointing.

Clonorchis infects man but otherwise resembles *Fasciola*. It may lead to cancer of the bile duct.

Tapeworms (cestodes)

Cestodes may live harmlessly in the intestine (e.g. **Taenia**), occasionally invading, and dying in, the brain ('cysticercosis'), or establish cystic colonies in the liver, etc. (e.g. the hydatid cysts of **Echinococcus**), where the worms are shielded from the effects of antibody. Antigen from the latter, if released (e.g. at surgery) can cause severe immediate hypersensitivity reactions (see Fig. 33).

31 Immunity to tumours

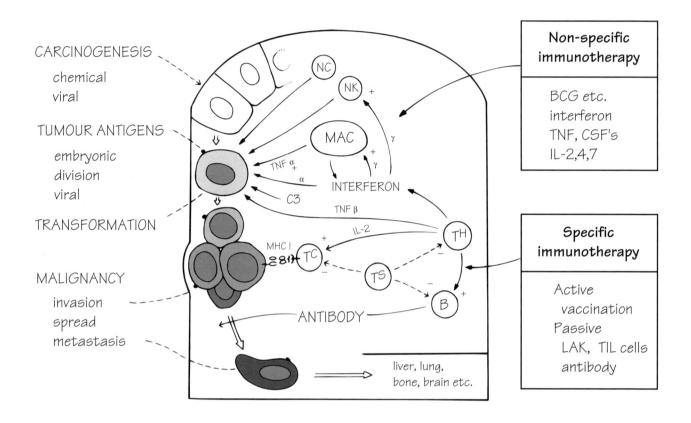

CARCINOGENESIS
- chemical
- viral

TUMOUR ANTIGENS
- embryonic
- division
- viral

TRANSFORMATION

MALIGNANCY
- invasion
- spread
- metastasis

Non-specific immunotherapy

BCG etc.
interferon
TNF, CSF's
IL-2,4,7

Specific immunotherapy

Active
  vaccination
Passive
  LAK, TIL cells
  antibody

liver, lung, bone, brain etc.

Immunologists have always hoped that when the 'conquest of cancer' is announced they will be among those sharing the credit, but it must be admitted that on present evidence this cannot be guaranteed. In its relationship to the host, a tumour cell (shaded in figure) is rather like a successful parasite, but with special additional features. Parasite-like mechanisms that may help prevent elimination include: **weak antigenicity** and extensive cross-reaction with self; **immuno-suppression**; release of **soluble antigens**; antigen–antibody **complexes**; and **antigenic variation**. Unlike parasites, however, spontaneous tumours are individually unique and usually of unknown origin, and they unfortunately lack the well-adapted parasite's sense of self-preservation through host-preservation (behaving more like virulent zoonoses). Moreover, apart from some childhood tumours, cancer occurs at too late an age to have had much selective effect on the evolution of immune defences. One could even argue that it is a useful way for a species to eliminate the aged and make room for the young.

Nevertheless, there are a few hopeful pointers. Most tumour cells *are* antigenic, albeit weakly, and experimental animals can often be specifically immunized against them. Immunodeficient and immunosuppressed patients do develop more tumours of certain tissues (though T cell-deprived mice do not). Cells that kill tumours *in vitro* can be isolated from both animals and humans with growing tumours, and rejection of secondary implants ('concomitant immunity'), can be found in animals with primary tumours. Most encouraging of all, tumours occasionally regress spontaneously, or after only partial destruction by surgery or chemotherapy.

As to which immune mechanisms are, or might be made, effective, opinion has swung away from all-embracing theories such as 'T cell surveillance' (which was an attempt to rationalize transplant rejection) towards the concept that different mechanisms, both natural (top) and adaptive (bottom), may work against different tumours—as they do against different infectious micro-organisms.

Carcinogenesis In mice, chemicals such as methylcholanthrene, benzpyrenes, etc. tend to induce tumours, each with unique 'idiotypic' antigens, whilst tumours induced by viruses, such as polyoma, Gross leukaemia, etc., share antigens characteristic of the virus. In humans, four viruses (all DNA) are firmly linked to tumours: EBV (Burkitt's lymphoma), CMV (Kaposi's sarcoma), HBV (hepatocarcinoma) and papilloma virus (cervical cancer), but RNA retroviruses, by activating the cell's own oncogenes, may be responsible for some other cases. Most of the common human cancers are probably not virally induced, but result from an accumulation of mutations in the genes of a variety of proteins which regulate the cell cycle. Such mutations can result in over-activation of a protein promoting cell growth (the genes encoding such proteins are known as *oncogenes*), or inactivation of a protein which normally slows down cell growth (the genes encoding such proteins are known as *tumour suppressor genes*). Sometimes some of these mutations are inherited, while others may result from exposure to chemicals in the environment. But normally, it requires several mutagenic events, which can occur over many decades, before a tumour develops.

Tumour antigens In the case of tumours induced by viruses, the **viral** antigens themselves can be the target of the host immune response. In non-viral tumours, the identification of tumour associated antigens (TAAs) has been much more difficult. In rare cases **Embryonic** antigens absent from normal adult cells may be re-expressed when they become malignant. Carcino-embryonic antigen (CEA) in the colon and α-fetoprotein in the liver are examples, of diagnostic value. Other antigens found on the surface of some tumours are glycosylation variants of normal cell proteins (e.g. MUC-1 on epithelial tumours). However, it seems that the majority of antigens recognized by the host's cellular immune response are normal self proteins, which are expressed at higher concentrations than normal in the tumour cells (sometimes because they are required for cell division). Examples are the specific idiotype of the antibody expressed on B cell lymphomas, or the 'stem-cell' antigen of acute lymphoblastic leukaemia.

Natural immunity

Mac, NK Macrophages and natural killer cells (see Fig. 9), especially when activated, can prevent growth of some tumours *in vitro* ('cytostasis') or actually kill them ('cytolysis'). Macrophage cytotoxicity may be mediated by release of TNF. NK cells are also cytotoxic, and are activated by cells which have lost expression of MHC molecules, a common phenotype of many tumours (see Fig. 9). IFNγ is important in activating macrophages and NK cells. Some tumour cells can apparently activate **complement** via the alternative pathway. This and the other mechanisms mentioned above may contribute to the surprising resistance of thymusless 'nude' mice to spontaneous tumours.

Adaptive immunity

Antibody There is little evidence that antibody normally provides any host immunity to tumours, although mice bred for high antibody responses have been reported to be more resistant to chemical carcinogenesis. It can sometimes actually 'enhance' tumour growth, probably by forming complexes with soluble antigens and blocking T cell-mediated cytotoxicity.

Cell-mediated immunity Cytotoxic CD8 T cells capable of lysing tumour cells *in vitro* have been isolated both from mice and humans (especially from individuals with melanoma). In mice such cytotoxic T cells can eliminate a tumour *in vivo*. Many tumours evade this by reducing their expression of MHC Class I antigens. T^H cells (of TH1 phenotype) are also probably very important, since they can activate macrophages and NK cells via the release of IFNγ. However, weak T cell reactions may actually stimulate tumour growth.

Suppression Suppressor T cells have been claimed to aid the growth of ultraviolet-induced skin cancer in mice, by inhibiting cytotoxic T cells. Patients with Burkitt's lymphoma carry high levels of EBV, and it has been suggested that tumours of the virus-infected B cells develop because of a suppression of the normally curative cytotoxic T cell response—malaria being the most likely cofactor.

Non-specific immunotherapy

BCG (an attenuated tubercle bacillus) has been tried against melanoma, sarcoma, etc., especially combined with other treatments. Its major immunological effect seems to be macrophage activation, but it may also affect NK cells. A tremendous range of bacterial and other immunostimulating agents is at present being tested for antitumour activity (see Fig. 41).

Cytokines The dramatic effects of 'Coley's toxin'—a bacterial extract—100 years ago may have been due to the vigorous induction of cytokines. A modern variant of this approach are current trials in which *Mycobacterium vaccae* is being used to induce protective antitumour immunity. Following the success of TNF in animals, numerous individual cytokines have also been tried on cancer patients. At present only IFNα and IL-2 are in widespread use, but improved delivery to the site of the tumour (for example by gene therapy) may extend this approach.

Specific immunotherapy

Vaccination with irradiated or enzyme-treated cells, cell hybrids, etc. can be very successful in animals before tumour induction. Clinical trials are in progress to see whether therapeutic immunization, using a variety of the TAAs discussed above, may be of value as an adjunct to chemotherapy or surgery. An alternative approach which is being tested initially for the treatment of melanoma, is to use tumour cells isolated from the patient, and then transfected with various cytokine genes to make the tumours more immunogenic. In the case of viral tumours, conventional vaccination to the viruses involved may be used to prevent subsequent development of cancer.

Passive administration of monoclonal antibodies to TAA is being tested in a variety of human tumours. In some cases, the antibody is used alone, harnessing the host's innate defence mechanism (e.g. complement and ADCC) to kill the tumour cells; this approach has had some remarkable successes in the treatment of cancer of the intestine, and of lymphoma. In other cases, the antibody is coupled to a cytotoxic drug, or to an enzyme which converts a prodrug into an active cytotoxic drug. This approach (named the 'magic bullet') aims to build up very high levels of anticancer drug, but only in the immediate vicinity of the tumour, thus minimizing the general toxicity of the drug which limits the concentrations which can normally be used for chemotherapy.

Lymphocytes Lymphocytes from the blood of tumour patients, activated *in vitro* by IL-2 (LAK cells), and lymphocytes extracted from the tumour itself (TIL cells), have in some cases been successful in causing tumour rejection.

32 Harmful immunity: a general scheme

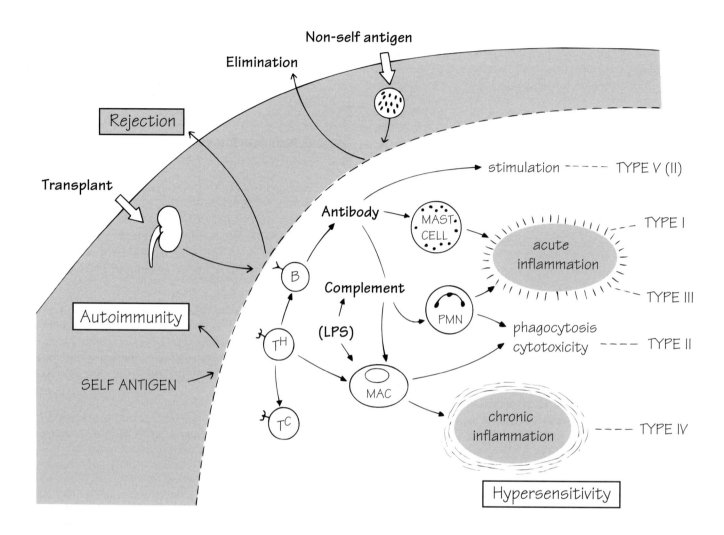

So far we have been considering the successful side of the immune system—its defence role against microbial infection (top). The effectiveness of this is due to two main features: (1) the wide range of antigens it can specifically recognize and remember, and (2) the strong non-specific mechanisms it can mobilize to eliminate them.

Unfortunately, both of these abilities can also operate against their possessor. (1) Wide-ranging specificity necessitates an efficient mechanism for avoiding action against 'self' determinants (bottom left: the problem of **autoimmunity**). Also there are cases where the elimination of non-self material may not be desirable (the problem of **transplant rejection**; top left). (2) Strong non-specific weapons (e.g. complement, polymorphs, macrophages and other inflammatory agents: centre) cannot always be trained precisely on the proper target, but may spill over to damage neighbouring tissues (the problem of **hypersensitivity**).

The nomenclature of these **immunopathological** reactions has never been very tidy. Originally any evidence of altered reactivity to an antigen

following prior contact was called 'allergy', while 'hypersensitivity', though intended for those effects which harmed the host, was in fact defined as 'acute', 'immediate', or 'delayed' on the basis of the time taken for changes—often quite innocuous skin test reactions—to appear. As knowledge grew, reactions could be classified according to the mechanism involved; this is the basis of the very influential scheme of Gell and Coombs (Types I to V; right), in which 'allergy' and 'hypersensitivity' retained their old meaning, but with the latter extended to include autoimmunity and transplant rejection. However, most immunologists now use 'allergy' in its everyday sense of immediate (Type I) hypersensitivity, e.g. to pollen. What is really needed is a separate word, without historical overtones, to cover those aspects for which specific recognition is not to blame (that is, excluding autoimmunity and transplant rejection). Meanwhile, it is safest to think in terms of both specific recognition *and* effector mechanisms when considering immunologically mediated tissue damage.

T^H Helper T cell, whose recognition of carrier determinants permits antibody responses by B cells and the activation of macrophages. There is little evidence that helper T cells ever react to absolutely unaltered 'self' antigens *in vivo* (but see Figs 22, 36).

B B lymphocyte, the potential antibody-forming cell. B lymphocytes that recognize many, though probably not all, 'self' determinants are found in normal animals; they can be switched on to make autoantibody by 'part-self' (or 'cross-reacting') antigens if a helper T cell can recognize a 'non-self' determinant on the same antigen (e.g. a drug or a virus; for further details see Fig. 36).

T^C Cytotoxic T cells against 'self' cells have been demonstrated in some autoimmune diseases (e.g. Hashimoto's hypothyroidism).

Mast cell A tissue cell with basophilic granules containing vasoactive amines, etc. which can be released following interaction of antigen with passively acquired surface antibody (IgE), resulting in rapid inflammation—local ('allergy') or systemic ('anaphylaxis'; see Fig. 33).

Complexes Combination with antigen is, of course, the basis of all effects of antibody. When there is an excess formation of antibody/antigen complexes, some of these settle out of blood onto the walls of the blood vessels (especially in the skin and kidneys). Tissue damage may then occur from the activation of complement, PMN, or platelets (see Fig. 34).

Complement is responsible for many of the tissue-damaging effects of antigen–antibody interactions, as well as their useful function against micro-organisms. The inflammatory effects are mostly due to the anaphylotoxins (C3a and C5a) which act on mast cells, while opsonization (by C3b) and lysis (by C5–9) are important in the destruction of transplanted cells and (via autoantibody) of auto-antigens.

PMN Polymorphonuclear leucocytes are attracted rapidly to sites of inflammation by complement-mediated chemotaxis, where they phagocytose antigen–antibody complexes; their lysosomal enzymes can cause tissue destruction, as in the classic Arthus reaction.

PL Platelets. Antigen-antibody complexes bind to and aggregate platelets, causing vascular obstruction as well as vasoactive amine release. Platelet aggregation is a prominent feature of kidney graft rejection.

MAC Macrophages are important in phagocytosis, but may also be attracted and activated, largely by T cells, to the site of antigen persistence, resulting in both tissue necrosis and granuloma formation (see Fig. 35). The slower arrival of monocytes and macrophages in the skin following antigen injection gave rise to the name 'delayed hypersensitivity'. Note that a number of microbial molecules can activate macrophages directly, for example the effect of bacterial endotoxin (**LPS**) in causing TNF and IL-1 release. When this occurs on a large scale, it can result in vascular collapse and damage to several organs. This 'endotoxin shock' is a feature of infections with meningococci and other Gram-negative bacteria. LPS can also directly activate the complement (alternative) and clotting pathways.

Types of hypersensitivity (Gell and Coombs classification)

I Acute (anaphylactive; immediate; reaginic): mediated by IgE and sometimes IgG antibody together with mast cells (e.g. hay fever).

II Antibody-mediated (cytotoxic): mediated by IgG or IgM together with complement, K cells or phagocytic cells (e.g. blood transfusion reactions; many autoimmune diseases). It could be argued that this is not 'true' hypersensitivity, since these examples can be equally well classified as autoimmunity or transplant rejection, but see also V below.

III Complex-mediated: inflammation involving complement, polymorphs, etc. (e.g. Arthus reaction; serum sickness; chronic glomerulonephritis).

IV Cell-mediated (delayed; tuberculin-type): T cell dependent recruitment of macrophages, eosinophils, etc. (e.g. tuberculoid leprosy; schistosomal cirrhosis; viral skin rashes; skin graft rejection).

V Stimulatory: a recent proposal to split off from Type II those cases where antibody directly stimulates a cell function (e.g. stimulation of the thyroid TSH receptor in thyrotoxicosis). For the sake of completeness, a place must also be found somewhere for the 'blocking' and 'enhancing' antibodies of tumour immunity, and for polyclonal B cell activation (e.g. in trypanosomiasis), both of which can undoubtedly be against the patient's best interests.

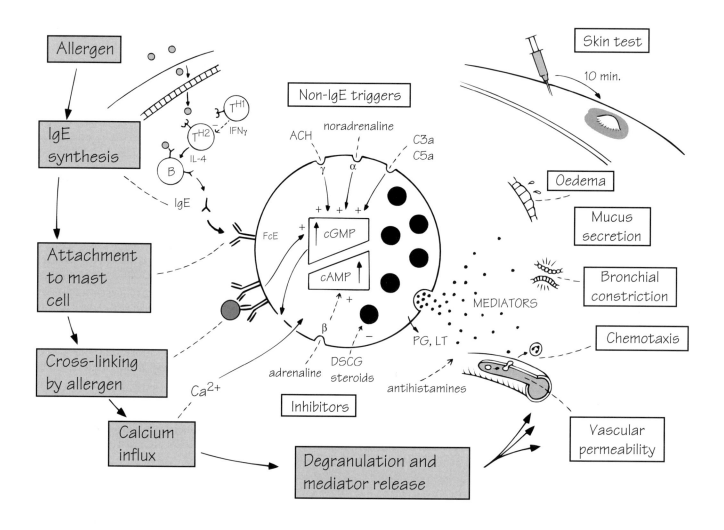

By far the commonest form of hypersensitivity is Gell and Coombs' Type I, which embraces such everyday **allergic** conditions as hay fever, eczema and urticaria but also the rare and terrifying **anaphylactic** reactions to bee stings, peanuts, penicillin, etc. In both cases the underlying mechanism is a sudden degranulation of **mast cells** with the release of inflammatory **mediators**, triggered by specific antibodies of the **IgE** class. It is therefore an example of acute inflammation (as already described in Fig. 6) but induced by the presence of a particular antigen rather than by injury or infection. With systemic release (anaphylaxis) there is bronchospasm, vomiting, skin rashes, oedema of the nose and throat, and vascular collapse, sometimes fatal, whilst with more localized release one or other of these symptoms predominates, depending on the site of exposure to the antigen.

Antigens that can trigger these reactions are known as 'allergens'. People who suffer unduly from allergy are called 'atopic'; this trait is usually inherited and has been attributed to a variety of constitutional abnormalities. Since worm antigens are among the most powerful allergens, the existence of this unpleasant and apparently useless form of immune response has been assumed to date from a time when worm infections were a serious evolutionary threat. Inflammation itself, of course, is an invaluable part of the response to injury and infection, and where injury is minimal (e.g. worms in the gut), IgE offers a rapid and specific trigger for increasing access of blood cells, etc., to the area.

There is a close link between inflammation and the emotions via the autonomic nervous system, through the influence of the sympathetic (α and β) and para-sympathetic (γ) receptors on intracellular levels of the cyclic nucleotides AMP and GMP, which in turn regulate cell function — in the case of mast cells, mediator release (see Fig. 24). Note also that mast cell degranulation can be triggered directly by tissue injury (see Fig. 6) and complement activation (see Fig. 34).

IgE The major class of reaginic (skin sensitizing; homocytotropic) antibody. Normally less than 1/10 000 of total Ig, its level can be up to 30 times higher, and specific antibody levels 100 times higher, in allergic or worm-infested patients. Binding of its Fc portion to receptors (Fcε) on mast cells and basophils, followed by cross-linking of adjacent molecules by antigen, triggers degranulation. Injection of antigen into the skin of allergic individuals causes inflammation within minutes—the 'immediate skin response'. Antigen responsiveness can be transferred to guinea-pigs by serum—the passive cutaneous anaphylaxis (PCA) test. IgG antibody, by efficiently removing antigens, can protect against mast cell degranulation. However, some IgG subclasses (in the human, IgG4) may have transient reaginic effects as well.

T^H Helper T cell. IgE production by B cells is dependent on the cytokine IL-4, released by T^{H2} cells. In atopic patients, allergens tend to induce an unbalanced production of the 'T^{H2} type' cytokines IL4, IL5, etc., and very little of the T^{H1} cytokines such as IFNγ which down regulate IgE production. There is also evidence for various other T cell derived factors that augment or reduce IgE production.

Mast cells in the tissues and blood **basophils** are broadly similar, but there are differences in the content of mediators. There are also important differences between the mast cells in the lung and gut ('mucosal') and those around blood vessels elsewhere ('connective tissue'). Mucosal mast cells are interesting in being regulated by (and according to some workers even derived from) T lymphocytes.

Eosinophils are believed to play an important role in inflammation in the lung, which can lead to asthma, and perhaps also to gut inflammatory diseases, including those which may underlie some food allergies. Like mast cells they release a variety of inflammatory mediators, and they too are regulated by T cell derived cytokines, especially IL-5.

Ca^{2+} Following the cross-linking of IgE receptors, membrane lipid changes lead to the entry of calcium, and an increase in adenylate cyclase, which in turn raises cAMP levels.

cAMP, cGMP Cyclic adenosine/guanosine monophosphates, the relative levels of which regulate cell activity. A fall in the cAMP/cGMP ratio is favoured by Ca^{2+} entry and by activation of α and γ receptors, and results in degranulation. Activation of the β receptor (e.g. by adrenaline) has the opposite effect; atopic patients may have a partial defect of β receptor function, permitting excessive mediator release.

Atopy is a condition characterized by high levels of circulating IgE antibodies, which predisposes the individual to the development of allergy. The development of atopy is regulated both by genetic and environmental factors, which are currently the object of intense study. The genetic regulation of atopy is complex and multigenic, involving polymorphisms at 20 or more loci. Interestingly, the prevalence of atopy is on the increase. This has been variously attributed to increased levels of pollutants in the environment, or, more convincingly, to decreased exposure to bacterial infection during early childhood, and hence an imbalance in the developing T^{H1}/T^{H2} balance of the immune system.

Mediators
Many of these are preformed in the mast cell granules, including **histamine**, which increases vascular permeability and constricts bronchi, **chemotactic** factors for neutrophils and eosinophils, and a factor which activates platelets to release their own mediators. Others are newly formed after the mast cell is triggered, such as prostaglandins (**PG**) and leukotrienes (**LT**; see Fig. 6 for details), which have similar effects to histamine but act less rapidly.

Inhibitors
SCG Sodium chromoglycate ('Intal'), and **steroids** (e.g. betamethasone) are thought to inhibit mediator release by stabilizing lysosomal membranes. Other drugs used in allergy include **antihistamines** (which do not, however, counteract the other mediators), **adrenaline**, isoprenaline, etc., which stimulate β receptors, anticholinergics (e.g. atropine), which block γ receptors, and theophylline, which raises cAMP levels. It has been gratifying to physicians to see the new molecular pharmacology of cell regulation confirming so many of their empirical observations on the control of allergic disease.

Non-IgE triggering
The complement products C3a and C5a can cause mast cells to degranulate, and so can some chemicals and insect toxins. Such non-IgE mediated reactions are called 'anaphylactoid'.

Allergic diseases
Originally the term 'atopy' referred only to hay fever and asthma, which are usually due to plant or animal 'allergens' in the air, such as pollens, fungi, and mites; it is still debatable whether all asthma is caused by allergy. However, similar allergens may also cause skin reactions (urticaria), either from local contact or following absorption. Urticaria after eating shellfish, strawberries, cow's milk, etc. is a clear case where the site of entry and the site of reaction are quite different, due to the ability of IgE antibodies to attach to mast cells anywhere in the body. There is mounting evidence for the role of food allergy in migraine and in other ill-defined physical and mental 'aches and pains'.

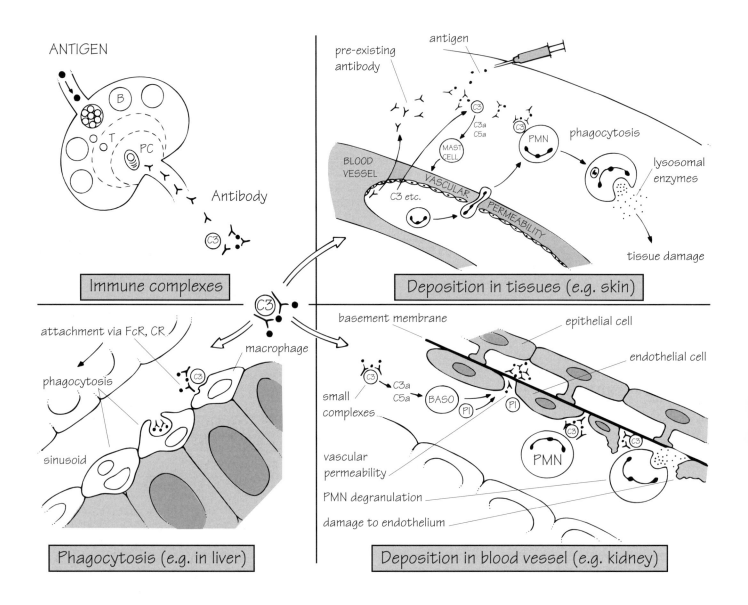

All the useful functions of antibody depend on its ability to combine with the corresponding antigen to form an **immune complex** (glance back at Fig. 19 to be reminded of the forces which bring this about). The normal fate of these complexes is phagocytosis (bottom left) which is greatly enhanced if complement becomes attached to the complex; thus complex formation is an essential prelude to antigen disposal.

However, there are circumstances when this fails to happen, particularly if the complexes are small (e.g. with proportions such as Ag2:Ab1; Ag3:Ab2). This can occur if there is an **excess** of antigen, as in persistent infections and in autoimmunity, or where the antibody is of very low affinity, or where there are defects of the phagocytic or the complement systems.

If not rapidly phagocytosed, complexes can induce serious inflamma-

tory changes in either the tissues (top right) or in the walls of small blood vessels (bottom right), depending on the site of formation. In both cases it is activation of **complement** and enzyme release by **polymorphs** which do the damage. The renal glomerular capillaries are particularly vulnerable, and immune complex disease is the commonest cause of chronic glomerulonephritis, which is itself the most frequent cause of kidney failure.

Note that increased vascular permeability plays a preparatory role both for complex deposition in vessels and for exudation of complement and PMN into the tissues, underlining the close links between Type I and Type III hypersensitivity. Likewise there is an overlap with Type II, in that some cases of glomerulonephritis are due to antibody against the basement membrane itself, but produce virtually identical damage.

Complexes of small size are formed in antigen excess, as occurs early in the antibody response to a large dose of antigen, or with persistent exposure due to drugs, chronic infections (e.g. streptococci, hepatitis, malaria), or associated with autoantibodies.

Macrophages lining the liver (Kupffer cells) or spleen sinusoids remove particles from the blood, including large complexes.

PMN Polymorphonuclear leucocyte, the principal phagocyte of blood, whose granules (lysosomes) contain numerous antibacterial enzymes. When these are released neighbouring cells are often damaged. This is particularly likely to happen when the PMN attempts to phagocytose complexes which are fixed to other tissues.

C3 The central component of complement, a series of serum proteins involved in inflammation and antibacterial immunity. C3 is split when complexes bind C1, C4 and C2, into a small fragment, C3a, which activates mast cells and basophils and a larger one, C3b, which promotes phagocytosis by attaching to receptors on PMN (and macrophages). Subsequent components generate chemotactic factors that attract PMN to the site. C3 can also be split via the 'alternative' pathway initiated by bacterial endotoxins, etc. Complement is also responsible for preventing the formation of large precipitates and solubilizing precipitates once they have formed (see also Fig. 5).

Mast cells, basophils, and **platelets** contribute to increased vascular permeability by releasing histamine, etc. (see Fig. 33).

The glomerular **basement membrane** (GBM), together with endothelial cells and external epithelial 'podocytes', separates blood from urine. Immune complexes are usually trapped on the blood side of the BM, except when antibody is directed specifically against the GBM itself (as in the autoimmune disease Goodpasture's syndrome) but small complexes can pass through the BM to accumulate in the urinary space. Mesangial cells may proliferate into the subendothelial space, presumably in an attempt to remove complexes. Endothelial proliferation may occur too, resulting in glomerular thickening and loss of function.

Immune complex diseases

The classic types of immune complex disease, neither of which is much seen nowadays, are the **Arthus reaction**, in which antigen injected into the skin of animals with high levels of antibody induces local tissue necrosis (top right in figure) and **serum sickness**, in which passively injected serum, for example a horse antiserum used to treat pneumonia, induces an antibody response, early in the course of which small complexes are deposited in various blood vessels, causing a fever with skin and joint symptoms about a week later. Certain diseases, however, are thought to represent essentially the same type of pathological reactions.

SLE Systemic lupus erythematosus, a disease of unknown, possibly viral, origin in which autoantibodies to nuclear antigens (which include DNA, RNA and DNA/RNA associated proteins) are deposited, with complement, in the kidney, skin, joints, brain, etc. Treatment is by immunosuppression or, in severe cases, exchange transfusion to deplete autoantibody.

Polyarteritis nodosa A disease of small arteries affecting numerous organs. Some cases may be due to complexes of hepatitis B antigen with antibody and complement.

RA Rheumatoid arthritis features both local (Arthus-type) damage to joint surfaces and systemic vasculitis. The cause is unknown but autoantibodies to IgG are a constant finding.

Alveolitis caused by *Actinomyces* and other fungi (see Fig. 28) may be due to an Arthus-type reaction in the lung.

Thyroiditis and perhaps other autoimmune diseases may be due to complex-mediated (i.e. autoantigen plus autoantibody) damage to the organ. With developments in the technique of detecting immune complexes (there are now over 20 different methods, see Fig. 19) it is likely that more diseases will be added to this list.

Infectious diseases The skin rashes and renal complications of several infections may be due to Type III reactions. In addition, widespread activation of complement can occur in septic shock, induced by LPS from Gram-negative bacteria, and in the haemorrhagic shock of viruses such as Dengue, in both of which it is associated with cytokines such as TNF. Complement, neutrophils, and cytokines are also thought to be involved in the pulmonary vascular leakage of the Adult Respiratory Distress Syndrome (ARDS) that follows massive trauma.

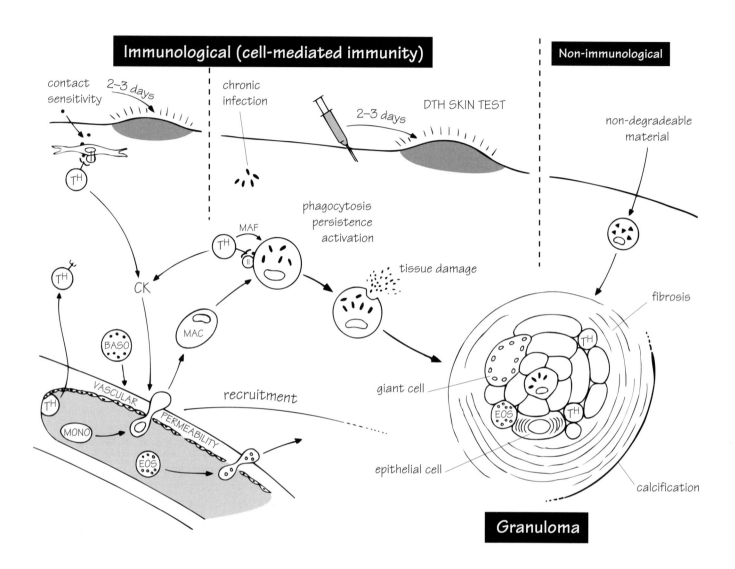

Following the changes in permeability, the activation of complement, and the influx of polymorphs, the last arrivals at sites of inflammation are the 'mononuclear cells': **lymphocytes** and **monocytes** (bottom left). Lymphocytes are usually specific in their attack, and only cause harm when attack is not called for (i.e. when the target is 'self' or a transplant), but monocytes and macrophages are equipped with enzymes which they normally use in the process of mopping up dead tissue cells and polymorphs, but which can also damage healthy cells, including other macrophages. When the stimulus is persistent, the result may be a growing mass of macrophages, or granuloma (bottom right), the hallmark of **chronic inflammation**.

These changes can occur in the absence of any specific immune response (e.g. reactions to foreign bodies; top right), but they are often greatly augmented by the activity of specific T lymphocytes (left) which,

by secreting cytokines, attract and immobilize monocytes and activate macrophages. When this process is predominantly beneficial (as in healed tuberculosis) we speak of '**cell-mediated immunity**' (CMI); when it is harmful (as in contact sensitivity or schistosomal cirrhosis) it is termed '**Type IV hypersensitivity**', the underlying pathology being the same and the difference one of emphasis (compare with Fig. 20). Confusingly, direct killing by cytotoxic T cells is also called 'cell-mediated immunity', though since it mainly affects virus-containing cells, a better name would be 'cell-mediated autoimmunity' or, in the case of organ grafts, 'cell-mediated transplant rejection'.

In any case, it is rare for one type of tissue damage to occur in isolation, interaction of cells and sharing of biochemical pathways being a feature of immune mechanisms, useful and harmful alike.

Cell-mediated immunity (CMI)

Contact between recirculating T cells and antigen leads to cytokine secretion with attraction and activation of monocytes and other myeloid cells (see Fig. 20 for further details). In the case of persistent antigens, particularly with intracellular infections such as tuberculosis, leprosy, brucellosis, leishmaniasis, schistosomiasis (the egg granuloma), trichinosis and fungi such as *Histoplasma*, chronic inflammation may result.

Delayed hypersensitivity (DTH)

The key feature of CMI is antigen-specific memory, which can be tested for *in vitro* by measuring lymphocyte proliferation or the release of cytokines such as IFNγ, or *in vivo* by the response to antigen injected into the skin. A positive DTH response consists of a reddened swelling 2–3 days later, the Mantoux test for tuberculosis being a typical example. While DTH frequently correlates with protective immunity, this is not invariably the case. Sometimes basophils are prominent, giving a quicker response known as 'Jones Mote' hypersensitivity.

Contact sensitivity

In this variant of DTH, antigens (usually plant or chemical molecules) become attached to antigen-presenting Langerhans cells in the skin, where T^H cells respond to them. The result is an eczema-like reaction with oedema and mononuclear cell infiltration 1–2 days later.

Chronic non-immunological inflammation

Materials which are phagocytosed but cannot be degraded, or which are toxic to macrophages, such as talc, silica, asbestos, cotton wool, some metals and their salts and bacterial products such as the cell wall peptidoglycan of group A streptococci, will give rise to granulomas even in T cell deprived animals, and are therefore considered to be able to activate (or 'anger') macrophages without the aid of T cells.

Granulomas

Granulomas are initiated and maintained by the recruitment of macrophages into the site where persistent antigen or toxic materials occur. Immune complexes are also a stimulus for granuloma formation.

Tissue damage may be caused by lysosomal enzymes released by macrophages, and perhaps by specialized cytotoxic molecules such as TNF.

Epithelioid cells are large cells found in palisades around necrotic tissue. They are thought to derive from macrophages, specialized for enzyme secretion rather than phagocytosis. There is some evidence that CMI favours their development.

Giant cells are formed by fusion of macrophages; they are particularly prominent in 'foreign-body' granulomas.

Eosinophils are often found in granulomas, perhaps attracted by antigen–antibody complexes, but also under the influence of T cells.

Fibrosis around a granuloma represents an attempt at 'healing'. Long-standing granulomas, i.e. healed tuberculosis, may eventually calcify, e.g. the well-known Ghon focus in the lung X-ray of many healthy people.

Granulomatous diseases

Granulomas are found in several diseases, some with a known aetiology, and some of unknown aetiology, suggesting an irritant or immunological origin. A few of the better-known are listed below.

Sarcoidosis is characterized by nodules in the lung, skin, eye, etc. An interesting feature is a profound deficiency of T cell immunity and often an increased Ig level and antibody responsiveness.

Crohn's disease (regional ileitis) is somewhat like sarcoidosis, but usually restricted to the intestine. It has been claimed that it is due to autoimmunity against gut antigens stimulated by cross-reacting bacteria. **Ulcerative colitis** may have a similar aetiology.

Temporal arteritis is a chronic inflammatory disease of arteries, with granulomas in which giant cells are prominent.

Primary biliary cirrhosis In this rare autoimmune disease (see also Fig. 36), granulomas form around the bile ducts. The disease is believed to result from cross-reaction between a bacterial antigen and a mitochondrial 'self-antigen'.

Eosinophilic granuloma Sometimes eosinophils outnumber the other cells in a granuloma; this is particularly seen in worm infections and in rare bone conditions.

Chronic granulomatous disease (CGD) An immunodeficiency disease, characterized by a defect in granulocyte function, which leads to chronic bacterial infection and granuloma development (see Fig. 39).

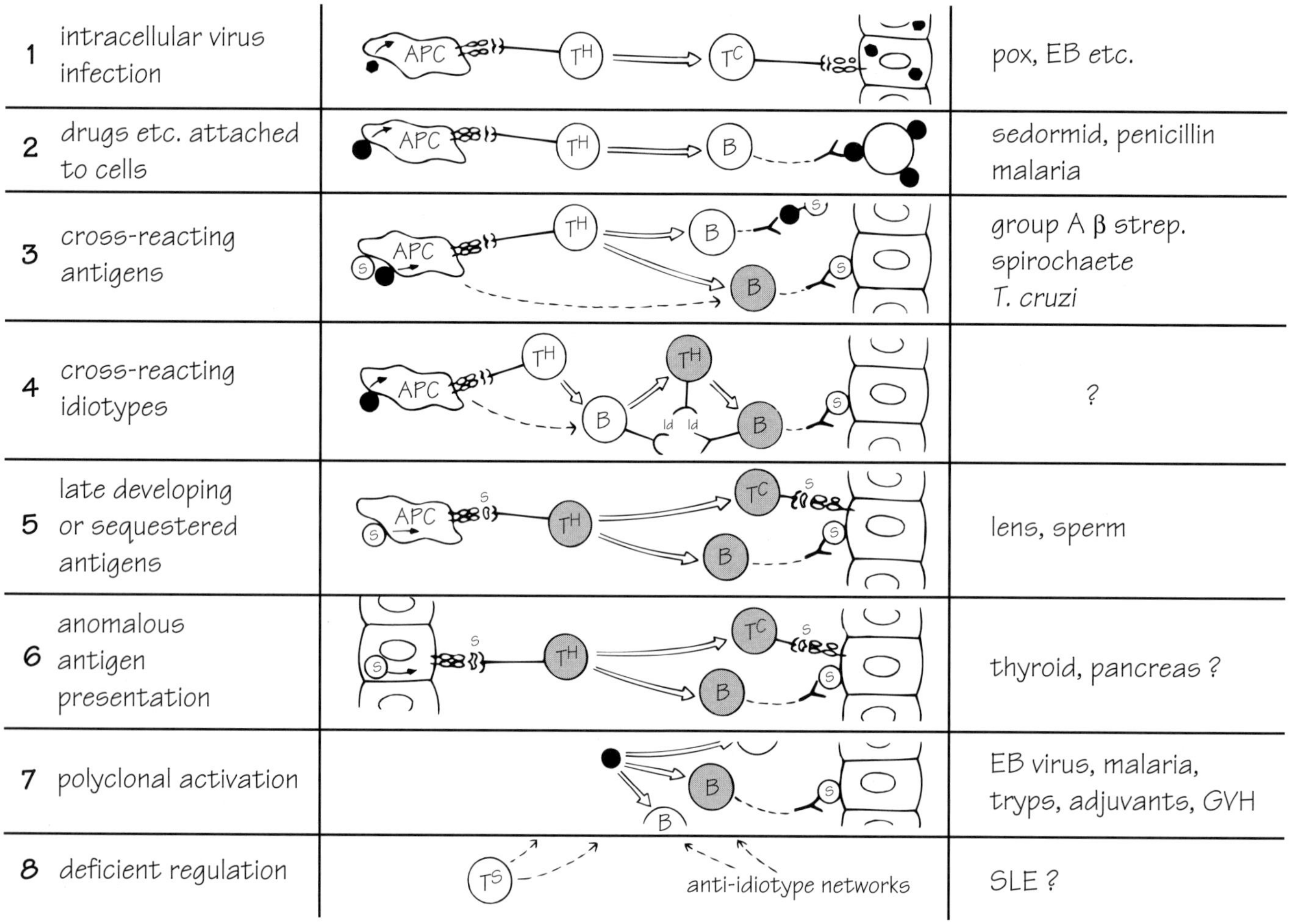

1	intracellular virus infection		pox, EB etc.
2	drugs etc. attached to cells		sedormid, penicillin malaria
3	cross-reacting antigens		group A β strep. spirochaete *T. cruzi*
4	cross-reacting idiotypes		?
5	late developing or sequestered antigens		lens, sperm
6	anomalous antigen presentation		thyroid, pancreas ?
7	polyclonal activation		EB virus, malaria, tryps, adjuvants, GVH
8	deficient regulation	anti-idiotype networks	SLE ?

Autoimmunity is the mirror image of tolerance, reflecting the *loss* of tolerance to 'self', and before proceeding, the reader is recommended to glance back at Fig. 21, which summarizes the mechanisms by which the immune system normally safeguards its lymphocytes against self-reactivity.

These mechanisms can be overcome in a number of ways, and it is quite illusory to look for a single cause of autoimmunity. In the figure, eight possible ways are shown, and often two or more of these may occur together. Sometimes a 'self' cell displaying 'non-self' antigens is unavoidably destroyed in the process of eliminating the intruder (lines 1 and 2; foreign antigens are shown in black throughout the figure and self-reactive lymphocytes shaded). Sometimes (lines 3 and 4) an invading organism sharing features with the host triggers off an antibody response against normal 'self' (S). For this to happen there must be some self-reactive B cells already present as explained in Fig. 21, clonal elimination of self-reactive cells is by no means complete for the B cells. Occasionally a 'self' antigen comes in contact with the immune system only at a late stage, when it is treated as 'non-self' (line 5).

Antigen presentation by cells not normally specialized for this role may give rise to self reactivity (line 6). Self-reactive B cells can be stimulated directly by 'polyclonal activators' which override the usual triggering requirements (line 7). And finally, any breakdown in the suppressor cell and anti-idiotype regulatory networks (line 8) is likely to allow autoimmune reactions to build up to the point where they can cause disease. Note that the old idea that autoantibodies were simply new 'mutant' antibodies is out of fashion because they are so seldom monoclonal, although it may still apply in particular cases.

Understanding of autoimmunity has been advanced by animal experiments, in particular: (a) the induction of autoantibody in normal animals by cross-reacting ('part-self') antigens, assumed to be due to co-operation between self-reactive B and non-self-reactive T cells (line 3), and (b) spontaneous autoimmune diseases in inbred strains of animals, notably the NZB mouse and the OS chicken, which reveal a multiplicity of genetic influences, at the level of B cells, T cell subsets, macrophages, target tissues, and hormones (autoimmunity is much commoner and more severe in females).

Induction of self-reactivity

Viruses, especially those which bud from cells (see Figs 20, 26), become associated with MHC Class I antigens and the combination is recognized by cytotoxic T cells. Other viruses such as influenza may attach to red cells and induce autoantibody.

Drugs frequently bind to blood cells, either directly (e.g. sedormid to platelets; penicillin to red cells) or as complexes with antibody (e.g. quinidine). The case of α-methyl dopa is different in that the antibodies are against cell antigens, usually of the Rhesus blood group system, towards which B cell tolerance is particularly unstable.

Cross-reacting antigens shared between microbe and host may stimulate T help for otherwise silent self-reactive B cells — the 'T cell bypass'. Cardiac damage in streptococcal infections and Chagas' disease appear to be examples of this. With the development of computer 'banks' of protein sequences, a number of self-antigens have been found to share significant amino acid sequences with viruses and bacteria, suggesting that abnormal responses to infection may be an important trigger in many autoimmune diseases.

Cross-reacting idiotypes This idea is based on the demonstration of (1) idiotype-specific T helper cells, and (2) idiotype sharing between antibodies of different specificity. It might explain the autoantibodies seen during infections (e.g. mycoplasma) which do not react with the organism.

Late developing (e.g. sperm) or **sequestered** (e.g. lens protein) **antigens** are assumed not to be 'seen' by lymphocytes until released by organ damage (e.g. eye injury; mumps orchitis).

Anomalous antigen presentation may occur when, possibly as a result of virus infection, Class II antigens are expressed on normal tissue cells. Thyroiditis is the best studied example so far, and IFNγ is suspected of being one of the triggering factors.

Polyclonal activation Many microbial products, e.g. endotoxins, DNA, etc., can stimulate B cells, including self-reactive ones. The Epstein–Barr virus infects B cells themselves and can make them proliferate continuously.

Deficient regulation is easy to visualize but hard to prove. There is claimed to be abnormally poor T suppressor function in SLE.

Genetics of autoimmunity Most autoimmune diseases have a genetic component, and much effort is being devoted to identifying the genetic 'risk factors' associated with particular autoimmune diseases. The strongest associations are those with specific alleles of the MHC class II genes (HLA-D region), providing further evidence that CD4+ T cells play an important role in the aetiology of these diseases. However, there are probably more than 20 other loci which contribute to an individual's propensity to develop a particular autoimmune disease.

Autoimmune diseases

Autoantibodies are found in every individual but rarely cause disease. In some diseases, raised autoantibody levels are clearly effect rather than cause (e.g. cardiolipin antibodies in syphilis). But in some diseases they are the first, major, or only detectable abnormality.

Haemolytic anaemia and **thrombocytopaenia**, though they can be due to drugs, are more often idiopathic. The correlation between autoantibody levels and cell destruction is not always very close, suggesting another pathological process at work.

Thyroiditis is one of the best candidates for 'primary' autoimmunity. There may be stimulation (thyrotoxicosis) by antibody against the receptor for pituitary TSH, or inhibition (myxoedema) by cell destruction, probably mediated by cytotoxic T cells and autoantibody. Anomalous expression of DR (HLA Class II) antigen is found in many cases.

Pernicious anaemia results from a deficiency of gastric intrinsic factor, the normal carrier for vitamin B12. This can be caused both by autoimmune destruction of the parietal cells (atrophic gastritis) and by autoantibodies to intrinsic factor itself.

Diabetes, Addison's disease (adrenal hypofunction) and other endocrine diseases are often found together in patients or families, suggesting an underlying genetic predisposition. The actual damage is probably mainly T cell mediated.

Myasthenia gravis, in which neuromuscular transmission is intermittently defective, is associated with autoantibodies to, and destruction, the postsynaptic acetylcholine receptors. There are often thymic abnormalities and thymectomy may be curative, though it is not really clear why.

Rheumatoid arthritis is characterized by, and may be due to, autoantibody against IgG (rheumatoid factor). Joint damage may be partly mediated via immune complexes, but T cell dependent activation of macrophages to release TNF-α and IL-1 (Type IV hypersensitivity) is probably the main pathology.

SLE In systemic lupus erythematosus the autoantibodies are against nuclear antigens, including DNA, RNA and nucleic acid binding proteins. The resulting immune complex deposition is widespread throughout the vascular system, giving rise to a 'non-organ-specific' pattern of disease. Like the 'organ specific' diseases (above), non-organ specific diseases tend to occur together. It is not clear why different complexes damage different organs; a localizing role for the antigen itself is an obvious possibility.

Treatment of autoimmunity

No cures exist for most autoimmune diseases, and treatment is symptomatic; examples are anti-inflammatory drugs for rheumatoid arthritis, or insulin for Type I diabetes. Remarkable improvement in patients with rheumatoid arthritis has been achieved by treatment with a high affinity antibody against TNFα, which presumably blocks the inflammatory cascade within the joint: this remains the only example of a successful therapy using an anticytokine antibody. More antigen specific approaches to immuno-modulation which are currently being tested are vaccination against particular families of T cell receptors, or induction of oral tolerance by feeding autoantigens (see Fig. 38).

37 Transplant rejection

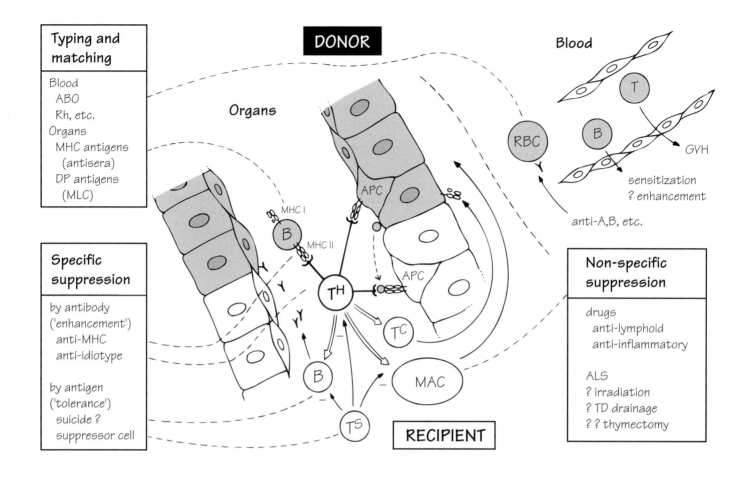

The success of organ grafts between identical ('syngenic'*) twins, and their rejection in all other cases, reflects the remarkable strength of immunological recognition of cell-surface antigens within a species. This is an unfortunate (and in the evolutionary sense unforeseeable) result of the specialization of T cells for detecting **alterations of MHC antigens**, upon which all adaptive responses depend (see Figs 18 and 20 for a reminder of the central role of T helper cells), plus the enormous degree of **MHC polymorphism** (different antigens in different individuals; see Fig. 13). It appears that when confronted with 'non-self' MHC molecules, T cells confuse them with 'self plus antigen', and in most cases probably 'self plus virus'; several clear examples of this have already been found in mouse experiments. This is probably the clue to MHC polymorphism itself: the more different varieties of 'self' a species contains, the less likely is any particular virus to pass undetected and decimate the whole species. Differences in red cell ('blood group') antigens also give trouble in blood transfusion (top right) because of antibody; here the rationale for polymorphism is less obvious, but it is much more restricted (e.g. six ABO phenotypes compared with over 10^{12} for MHC). The 'minor' histocompatibility and blood-group antigens appear to be both less polymorphic and antigenically weaker.

Graft rejection can be mediated by T and/or B cells, with their usual non-specific effector adjuncts (complement, cytotoxic cells, macrophages, etc.), depending on the target: antibody destroys cells free in the blood, and reacts with vascular endothelium (e.g. of a grafted organ: centre) to initiate Type III inflammation, while T cells attack solid tissue directly or via macrophages (Type IV). Unless the recipient is already sensitized to donor antigens, these processes do not take effect for a week or more, confirming that rejection is due to *adaptive*, not *natural* immunity.

Successful organ grafting relies at present on (top left) matching donor and recipient MHC antigens as far as possible (relatives and especially siblings are more likely to share these), and (bottom right) suppressing the residual immune response. The ideal would be (bottom left) to induce specific unresponsiveness to MHC antigens, but this is still experimental (see Fig. 38).

* Terminology: *syngenic, syngraft*: between genetically identical individuals; *allo-*(formerly *homo-*) non-identical, within species; *xeno-*between species; *auto-*same individual.

Typing and matching

For blood transfusion, the principle is simple: **A** and/or **B** antigens are detected by agglutination with specific antisera; this is always necessary because normal individuals have antibody against whichever antigen they lack. **Rh** (rhesus) antigens are also typed to avoid sensitizing women to those which a prospective child might carry, since Rh incompatibility can cause serious haemolytic disease in the fetus. Minor antigens only cause trouble in patients sensitized by repeated transfusions. Other possible consequences of blood transfusion are **sensitization** against MHC antigens carried on B cells, and, in severely immunodeficient patients, **GVH** (graft-vs.-host) reactions by transfused T cells against host antigens. The latter is a major complication of bone-marrow grafting.

For organ (e.g. kidney) grafting, MHC antigens must be typed (as well as ABO). This was done using panels of specific antisera, but antibody typing is now gradually being replaced by DNA typing, in which haplotype is determined using PCR and allele specific pairs of primers. One big advantage of this system is that it can be automated. The success of kidney grafting is related to the degree of match, particularly Class II, but the results with relatives suggest that there are other 'minor' histocompatibility loci, which are still being identified.

Rejection

The initial event is the recognition of 'altered self' Class II antigens by T helper cells. This can occur either by direct contact with donor B cells or antigen presenting cells (shaded APC in figure) or via the uptake of soluble donor antigens (shaded circles) by the recipient's own APC. Following this, B cells, cytotoxic T cells and macrophages are all triggered into action; which response destroys the graft, depends on the organ in question. Some points of special interest are listed below:

Kidney graft rejection can be **immediate**, due to ABO mismatch or pre-existing anti HLA antibodies, **acute** (weeks to months) due to the immune response, or **chronic** (months to years) due to re-emergence of disease. Surprisingly, blood transfusion before grafting improves survival, perhaps by inducing enhancing antibodies against Class II donor antigens.

Bone marrow contains the haemopoetic stem cell, and is therefore required whenever it is necessary to replace the host haemopoeitic system (for example in some immunodeficiencies or after high dose chemotherapy). More recently, however, it has been shown that the growth factor G-CSF causes haemopoetic stem cells to come out of the bone marrow and enter the circulation. As a result, blood can be used in place of bone marrow, a procedure known as peripheral stem cell transplantation. Any haemopoetic grafts are vigorously rejected, and require strong immunosuppression. In addition, they can kill the host by GVH reaction, unless T cells are removed from the donor marrow. A special case, not subject to this problem, is where bone marrow is removed from an individual before treatment (e.g. chemotherapy) and then reintroduced into the same individual (autologous transplant) to replace the damaged haemopoetic system.

Liver grafts are not so strongly rejected, and may even induce a degree of tolerance. HLA typing is less important.

Endocrine organs survive unexpectedly well if cultured or otherwise treated to remove the minority of cells expressing Class II antigens.

Skin grafts are rejected very vigorously by T cells, perhaps because of their extensive vascularization. For this reason, skin transplantation is usually either autologous, or a temporary graft used to protect the underlying tissue while the host's own skin regenerates (for example after extensive burns).

Cornea and **cartilage**, being non-vascular tissues, do not normally immunize the host and are allowed the 'privilege' of survival.

The normal **fetus** is of course an allograft, and why it is not rejected is still something of a mystery, despite evidence for a number of possible mechanisms, including specific suppressor cells, serum blocking and immunosuppressive factors, and special properties of both placenta (maternal) and trophoblast (fetal).

Xenografts There is considerable interest in the possibility of using animal donors for organ transplantation because of the continuing shortfall of available human organs. The pig is a suitable species for this because its size is comparable to a human. However, pig xenografts are rejected in primates within minutes by a process of hyperacute rejection. This is due to a combination of preformed antibodies against carbohydrate structures found in pigs but not primates, and the fact that the complement regulating proteins on pig tissue (e.g. DAF, see Fig. 5) do not interact well with human complement. Although attempts are being made to overcome these problems by introducing human genes into pigs, there is also continuing concern that pigs may harbour novel retroviruses, which could 'jump' the species barrier during transplantation and cause a new epidemic like AIDS.

Immunosuppression (see Fig. 38 for further details)

Non-specific The success of modern transplantation surgery is due largely to the introduction of cyclosporin, and later K506, two drugs which selectively block the activation of T cells in an antigen non-specific way (see Fig. 14). These two drugs, together with some cytotoxic drugs, are used at high concentrations postoperatively to block the initial acute rejection, and then at lower maintenance doses to block chronic rejection.

ALS Anti-lymphocyte serum, sometimes used in the hope of avoiding damage to dividing non-lymphoid cells (bone marrow; gut). Monoclonal antibodies to the CD4 antigen have been proposed as an alternative, although their efficacy in the clinic is still unclear.

TD (thoracic duct) drainage and **thymectomy** are occasionally used to deplete T cells.

Irradiation Total-body X-irradiation is highly immunosuppressive, and local irradiation (e.g. of a kidney) or extracorporeal irradiation of blood to destroy lymphocytes, are sometimes used in acute rejection crises.

Specific suppression is directed at either the antigens inducing a response or the receptors on the cells carrying it out. When brought about by antibody, this is conventionally called **enhancement** and when by antigen, **tolerance**. Antigen specific suppression is the goal of transplantation immunologists, but has still to be demonstrated in humans.

Suicide of specific T and B cells can be induced *in vitro* by letting them bind lethal (e.g. radioactive or drug-coupled) antigen.

Suppressor cells or antibodies, by mimicking normal 'network' control, might lead to stable tolerance, though this has not yet been achieved in man.

38 Immunosuppression

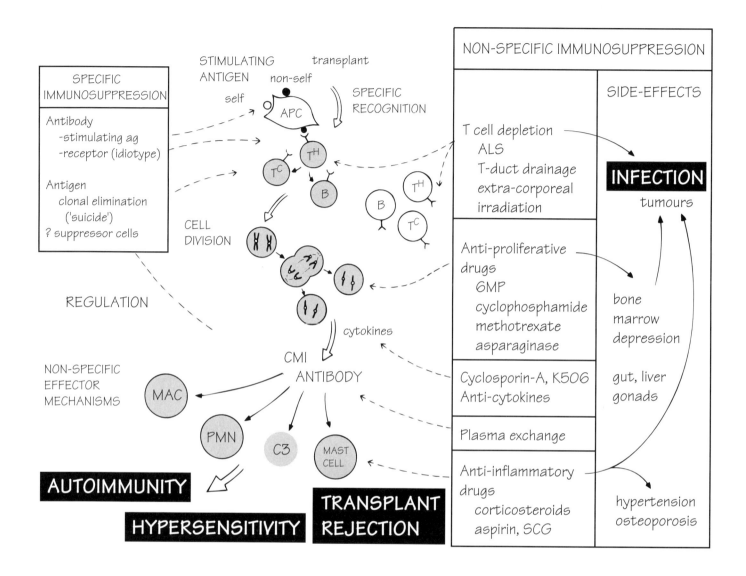

Suppression of immune responses, a regular part of the management of organ transplantation, can also be of value in cases of severe hypersensitivity and autoimmunity. Most of the methods currently available are more or less non-specific, and their use is limited by dangerous side-effects (right-hand side of figure).

The problem is to interfere with specific T and/or B cells (top centre, shaded) or their effects, without causing damage to other vital functions. T cells can be **depleted** by antilymphocyte antisera (ALS) and by removing or damaging recirculating cells (which are mostly T); however, this will remove not only undesirable lymphocytes but others upon whose normal response to infection life may depend (**B, T** unshaded). Lymphocytes almost always divide in the course of responding to antigen (centre), so drugs which inhibit **cell division** are effective immunosuppressants (the same drugs tend to be useful in treating cancer for the same reason); here the danger is that other dividing tissues, such as bone marrow and intestinal epithelium, will also be inhibited. A third point of attack is the **non-specific effector mechanisms** involved in the 'inflammatory' pathways (bottom) which so often cause the actual damage, but here again useful and harmful elements are knocked out indiscriminately.

What is clearly needed is an attack focused on antigen-specific lymphocytes—that is, an attack via their receptors (top left). This might take the form of masking the antigens they are stimulated by, masking or removing the receptors themselves, or using them to deliver a 'suicidal' dose of antigen to the cell. Whether any of these experimental approaches will be effective enough to replace the present clumsy but well-tried methods of immunosuppression, time will tell.

Non-specific immunosuppression

ALS (antilymphocyte serum) is made by immunizing horses or rabbits with human lymphocytes and absorbing out unwanted specificities. It depletes especially T cells, probably largely by opsonizing them for phagocytosis. It has found a limited use in organ transplantation. Monoclonal antibodies to particular T cell subsets or surface molecules, such as CD4, may have a more useful future.

Extracorporeal irradiation of blood, and **thoracic duct drainage** are drastic measures to deplete recirculating T cells, occasionally used in transplant rejection crises.

6MP (6-mercaptopurine) and its precursor **azathioprine** (Imuran) block purine metabolism, which is needed for DNA synthesis; despite side-effects on bone marrow polymorph and platelet production, they were for many years standard therapy in organ transplantation and widely used in autoimmune diseases, for example rheumatoid arthritis and SLE.

Cyclophosphamide and **chlorambucil** are 'alkylating' agents, which cross-link the DNA strands and prevent them replicating properly. Cyclophosphamide tends to affect B cells more than T, and there is some evidence that it also acts on Ig receptor renewal. It is effective in autoimmune diseases where antibody is a major factor (rheumatoid arthritis, SLE), but the common side-effect of sterility limits its use to older patients.

Methotrexate, fluorodeoxyuridine, and **cytosine arabinoside** are other examples of drugs inhibiting DNA synthesis by interfering with various pathways, which have been considered as possible immunosuppressives.

Asparaginase, a bacterial enzyme, starves dividing lymphocytes (and tumour cells) of asparagine, bone marrow, etc. being spared.

Cyclosporin A and K506 are important immunosuppressive agents obtained from fungi. They bind to intracellular molecules called immunophilins, and in doing so block activation of the T cell specific transcription factor NFAT, and hence the production of cytokines such as IL-2. Both have proved remarkably effective in bone marrow transplantation and have become the drug of choice for most transplants, although long-term use is associated with a risk of kidney damage. Cyclosporin has the added advantage of killing a number of micro-organisms, which might otherwise infect the immunosuppressed host. Other ways of blocking cytokines are also being tried, for example the use of soluble receptors or anticytokine antibodies.

Plasma exchange in which blood is removed and the cells separated from the plasma, and returned in dextran or some other plasma substitute, has been successful in acute crises of myaesthenia gravis and Goodpasture's syndrome by reducing (usually only transiently) the level of circulating antibody or complexes. It is also life-saving in severe rhesus disease of the newborn.

Corticosteroids (e.g. cortisone, prednisone) are, together with cyclosporin the mainstay of organ transplant immunosuppression, and are also valuable in almost all hypersensitivity and autoimmune diseases. They may act on T cells, but their main effect is probably on polymorph and macrophage activity. Sodium retention ($\rightarrow$ hypertension) and calcium loss ($\rightarrow$ osteoporosis) are the major undesirable side-effects.

Aspirin, indomethacin, SCG and a variety of other anti-inflammatory drugs are useful in autoimmune diseases with an inflammatory component (see Fig. 33 for other ways to control Type I hypersensitivity).

Specific immunosuppression

Regardless of the underlying mechanism, specific suppression mediated by antibody is traditionally known as 'enhancement' and that induced by antigen as 'tolerance'; however, since injection of antigen may often work by inducing antibody, both terms are better replaced, whenever possible, by a description of what is actually happening.

Antibody against **target antigens**, which is especially effective in preventing rejection of tumours, probably works by blocking Class II determinants, which may also be how blood transfusion improves kidney graft survival (see Fig. 37). Anti-rhesus (D) antibodies will prevent sensitization of Rh-negative mothers by removing the Rh-positive cells.

Antibody against receptor idiotypes, both B and T, might theoretically block recognition of antigen. Whether this block would be self-maintaining enough to be useful in transplantation or autoimmunity is uncertain.

Antibody against the CD4 molecule on T cells, when administered at the same time as antigen, seems to induce a state of long-lasting, antigen specific tolerance, at least in animal models. A similar approach is being tried for prevention of transplant rejection in humans.

Antigen administered over a prolonged period in very low doses can induce antigen-specific tolerance. This approach, known as desensitization, has long been used for the suppression of allergies.

Antigen administered via the oral (and perhaps also nasal) route induces strong antigen specific suppression in animals. A similar approach is being used in the treatment of autoimmune diseases; in one such trial patients with multiple sclerosis, in which autoimmune T cells attack the CNS, were fed extracts of animal myelin. The trial demonstrated a small therapeutic effect.

Clonal elimination, or 'classical tolerance' can be induced *in vitro* by coupling cytotoxic drugs or radio-isotopes to antigen, which is then concentrated on the surface of those cells specifically binding it; some success has also been obtained *in vivo* with this 'retiarian therapy' (named after Roman warriors who caught their victim with a net and then killed him with a spear). It is quite possible that the suppression caused by antiproliferative drugs (e.g. cyclophosphamide, cyclosporin A) in the presence of antigen, contains an element of specific clonal elimination.

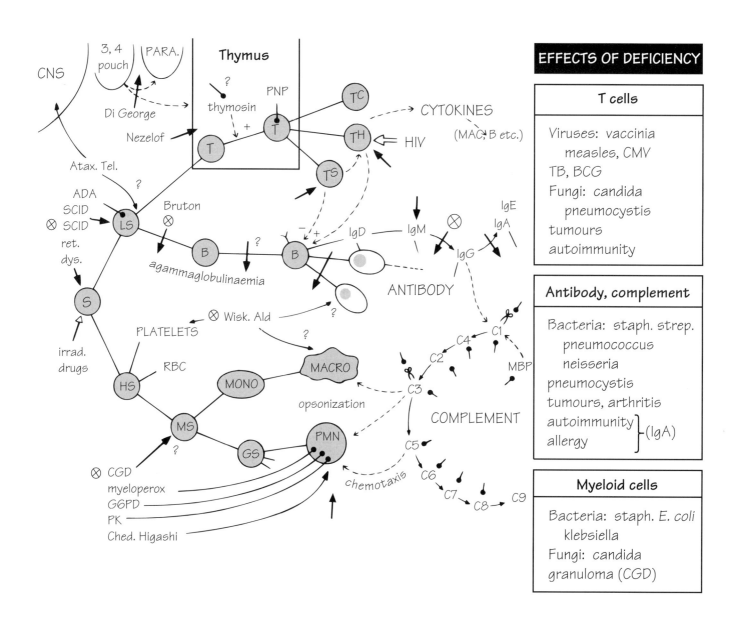

EFFECTS OF DEFICIENCY

T cells

Viruses: vaccinia
measles, CMV
TB, BCG
Fungi: candida
pneumocystis
tumours
autoimmunity

Antibody, complement

Bacteria: staph. strep.
pneumococcus
neisseria
pneumocystis
tumours, arthritis
autoimmunity }
allergy } (IgA)

Myeloid cells

Bacteria: staph. *E. coli*
klebsiella
Fungi: candida
granuloma (CGD)

Satisfactory immunity depends on the interaction of such an enormous variety of cells and molecules that inevitably a corresponding variety of different **defects** can reduce its efficiency, all with much the same end-result: increased susceptibility to infection (right). There is a tendency for somewhat different patterns of disease according to whether the defect predominantly affects T cells (top), antibody and/or complement (centre) or myeloid cells (bottom).

Immunodeficiency may be **secondary** to other conditions (e.g. drugs, malnutrition, or infection itself), or less commonly due to **primary** genetic defects. It is remarkable how many of the latter are 'X-linked' (i.e. inherited by boys from their mothers; in figure), suggesting that the unpaired part of the X chromosome carries several immunologically important genes. In some cases it appears that cell differentiation is interrupted at a particular stage (black arrows), but much more often there

is a variable mixture of partial and apparently disconnected defects. In an increasing number of diseases the missing gene product has now been identified (e.g. individual complement components, polymorph or lymphocyte enzymes (black circles), or cytokine receptor and adhesion molecules). Treatments being developed focus on replacement therapy, either using genes (gene therapy) or proteins,

The incidence of immunodeficiency depends on the definition of normality. Some form of obvious deficiency is found in more than one person per 1000, but this is clearly an underestimate, judging by the frequency with which 'normal' people succumb periodically to colds, sore throats, boils, etc. In fact the immunological basis of *minor* ill-health is a field whose surface has hardly been scratched.

(For details of cellular development and nomenclature, see Figs 4 and 9.)

Defects affecting several types of cell

Ret. dys   Reticular dysgenesis, a complete failure of stem cells, not compatible with survival for more than a few days after birth.

SCID   Severe combined immunodeficiency, in which both T and B cells are defective. Some cases are X-linked, and others appear to be due to deficiency of an enzyme, adenosine deaminase (**ADA**), which can be replaced by blood or marrow transfusion. Recent gene therapy trials in which recombinant retroviruses have been used to introduce the missing gene into bone marrow stem cells have shown some promise. In some cases, HLA Class I or II molecules are absent from lymphocytes ('bare lymphocyte syndrome').

Atax. Tel.   Ataxia telangectasia, a combination of defects in brain, skin, T cells and immunoglobulin (especially IgA), apparently due to a deficiency of DNA repair.

Wisk. Ald   Wiskott–Aldrich syndrome, another strange combination with eczema, platelet deficiency and absent antibody response to polysaccharides. The genetic defect for this disease is known to be in a protein which regulates cytoskeleton function, but how this results in the specific pathology observed remains unclear.

Defects predominantly affecting T cells

Di George syndrome; absence of thymus and parathyroids, with maldevelopment of other third and fourth pharyngeal pouch derivatives. Serious but very rare; it may respond to thymus grafting.

Nezelof syndrome; somewhat similar to Di George but with normal parathyroids and sometimes B cell defects.

PNP   Purine nucleoside phosphorylase, a purine salvage enzyme found in T cells. Deficiency causes nucleosides, particularly deoxyguanosine, to accumulate and damage the T cell. Interestingly, at low concentrations of deoxyguanosine, suppressor T cells are more sensitive than other types.

Cytokine defects, or defects in their receptors, appear to be rare, but IL-2 deficiency has been reported, as have individuals with deficiencies in the IL-12 receptor, and hence an inability to mount T^{H1} responses. There are also rare defects in many of the leucocyte adhesion molecules.

Defects predominantly affecting B cells

Agammaglobulinaemia or hypogammaglobulinaemia may reflect the absence of B cells (Bruton type), their failure to differentiate into plasma cells (variable types), or selective inability to make one class of immunoglobulin—most commonly IgA, but sometimes IgG or IgM. In X-linked hyper IgM syndrome, there is a genetic defect in the CD40 ligand molecule on T helper cells, which results in an inability to switch from making IgM to IgG.

Autoimmunity, allergies, and polyarthritis, are remarkably common in patients with antibody deficiencies, while both T and B cell defects appear to increase the risk of tumours (see Fig. 31).

Defects of complement

Virtually all the complement components may be genetically deficient; sometimes there is complete absence, sometimes a greatly reduced level, suggesting a regulatory rather than a structural gene defect. In addition, deficiency of inactivators may cause trouble, for example C1 inhibitor (hereditary angio-oedema); C3b inhibitor (very low C3 levels). In general, defects of C1, 4, 2 predispose to immune complex disease particularly SLE, and of C5–9 to neisserial infection. C3 deficiency, as expected (see Fig. 5) is the most serious of all, and seldom compatible with survival. Low levels of mannose-binding protein (**MBP**) predispose to severe infections in children.

Defects affecting myeloid cells

CGD   Chronic granulomatous disease, an X-linked defect of the oxygen breakdown pathway (see Fig. 8) usually involving a cytochrome, which leads to chronic infection with bacteria that do not themselves produce peroxide (catalase positive) and with fungi such as *aspergillus*. In a minority of cases there is another, non-X-linked, defect.

Myeloperoxidase, G6PD (glucose-6-phosphate dehydrogenase), **PK** (pyruvate kinase) and no doubt other polymorph enzymes may be genetically deficient, causing recurrent infection with bacteria and sometimes fungi.

Ched. Higashi   In the Chediak–Higashi syndrome, the polymorphs contain large granules but do not form proper phagolysosomes. In other cases the response to chemotaxis is impaired ('lazy leucocyte').

Secondary immunodeficiency

Age   Immunity tends to be weaker in infancy and old age—the former being partly compensated by passively transferred maternal antibody.

Malnutrition is associated with defects in antibody and, in severe cases, T cells; this may explain the more serious course of diseases (e.g. measles) in tropical countries. Both calorie and protein intake are important, as well as vitamins and minerals such as iron, copper and zinc.

Drugs can cause immunodeficiency, either intentionally (see Immunosuppression, Fig. 38) or unintentionally.

Infections   Immunosuppression is found in a great variety of infections, being one of the major parasite 'escape' mechanisms (see Figs 25–30). **HIV** infection, by progressively destroying CD4 T cells, weakens the whole immune system (see Fig. 40 for more about AIDS). Other viruses, such as measles, can temporarily depress T cell function. In all cases of T cell deficiency, cell-mediated responses are of course reduced, but there are often secondary effects on antibody as well.

Tumours are often associated with immunodeficiency, notably Hodgkin's disease, myeloma and leukaemias; it is sometimes hard to be sure which is cause and which effect.

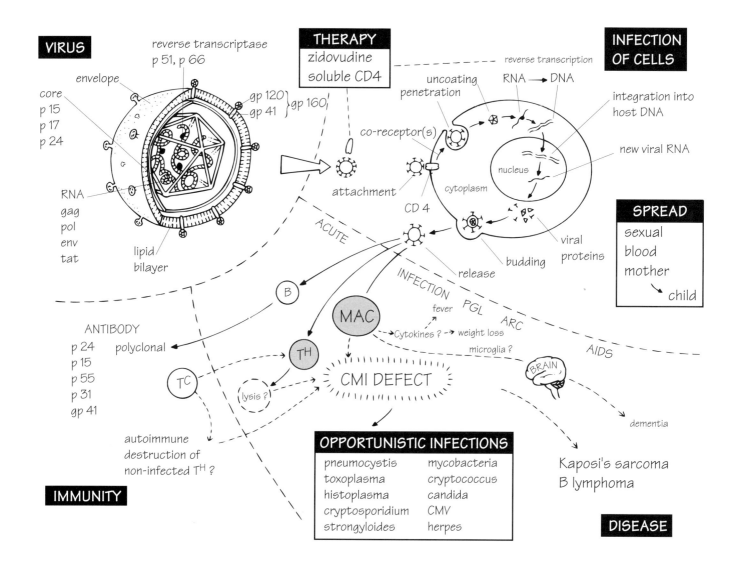

When in the summer of 1981 the American Centers for Disease Control noticed an unusual demand for a drug used to treat *Pneumocystis* pneumonia, a rare infection except in severely immunosuppressed patients, and cases began to be increasingly reported in homosexual men, haemophiliacs receiving certain batches of blood products, and drug users sharing needles, it became clear that a potentially terrible new epidemic had hit mankind, more insidious than the plague, more deadly than leprosy. The disease was baptized acquired immune deficiency syndrome (AIDS), and has become the most widely studied infectious disease of all time.

By 1984 the cause had been traced to a virus, now named HIV (human immunodeficiency virus), an RNA retrovirus which possesses the enzyme reverse transcriptase. This allows it to copy its RNA into DNA which is then integrated into the nucleus of the cells it infects, principally T helper cells and macrophages. By processes not fully understood, this leads to a slow disappearance of T helper cells, with derangement of the whole immune system and the development of life-threatening opportunistic infections and tumours.

HIV also possesses a number of other genes that give it an unusual ability to vary its antigens, which makes protective immunity or vaccination almost impossible to attain, and also to be stimulated by other viruses and cytokines. The latter has given rise to the suspicion that 'cofactors' may be required for the full development of AIDS.

HIV I and II, the AIDS viruses, closely related to the simian (monkey) virus SIV and more distantly to other retroviruses such as HTLV I and II which are rare causes of T cell leukaemias. Its genome consists of double-stranded RNA.

Gag The gene for the core proteins p17, p24, p15.

Pol The gene for various enzymes, including the all important reverse transcriptase.

Env The gene for the envelope protein gp160, which is cleaved during viral assembly to make gp120, the major structural protein of the viral envelope. This interacts initially with the **CD4** molecule found mainly on T cells and macrophages, but a second interaction with a member of the chemokine receptor family is required to allow the virus to infect cells. Different HIV strains interact preferentially with either the CCR5 receptor, found predominantly on macrophages, or the CXCR4 receptor found predominantly on activated T cells. About 1 in 10000 Caucasian individuals have a homozygous deletion in the CCR5 receptor, and these individuals are highly resistant to infection with HIV. Gag, pol, and env genes are found in all retroviruses.

Tat, rev, vif, nef genes unique to HIV, which can either enhance or inhibit viral synthesis.

Reverse transcriptase is required to make a DNA copy of the viral RNA. This may then be integrated into the cell's own nuclear DNA, from which further copies of viral RNA can be made, leading to the assembly of complete virus particles which bud from the surface to infect other cells. A key feature of this enzyme is that it allows errors in transcription to occur (on average there is one base pair mutation for every round of viral replication). This feature allows the rapid evolution of new variants of virus during the course of an infection.

Acute infection A few weeks after HIV infection some patients develop a glandular fever-like illness, though over 80% are symptomless.

Asymptomatic period Within a few weeks of infection, virus in the blood falls to very low levels, and remains low for variable periods between a few months and more than 20 years. During this period infected individuals show few symptoms, although the number of CD4+ T cells falls gradually. Despite this apparent 'latency', virus is in fact replicating rapidly and continuously, mainly within lymph nodes, and there is an enormous turnover of CD4+ T cells, as infected cells die and are replaced.

Symptomatic period Patients develop a variety of symptoms, including recurrent Candida, night sweats, oral hairy leukoplakia and peripheral neuropathy.

AIDS The full pattern includes the above plus severe life-threatening opportunistic infections and/or tumours. In some patients cerebral symptoms predominate. Estimates of the number of HIV-infected patients who will progress to AIDS vary from 50 to 100%, but it must be remembered that the disease is a slow one and has only been recognized for 20 years. The interval between infection and the development of progressive disease is very variable. It can be as short as 18 months, while in contrast some individuals remain healthy apparently

indefinitely. In 1998 there were estimated to be 33.4 million individuals infected with HIV/AIDS worldwide, of which 890000 were in North America, 500000 in Western Europe, and 32000 in the UK. In some countries (e.g. India) it seems that the AIDS epidemic has only recently begun.

Kaposi's sarcoma A disseminated skin tumour thought to originate from the endothelium of lymphatics. It is believed to be caused by human herpes virus-8(HHV-8), although it is still not clear why it is commoner in AIDS than in other immunodeficient conditions.

T cells are the most strikingly affected cells; the numbers of CD4+ (helper) T cells falling steadily as AIDS progresses, which leads to a failure of all types of T-dependent immunity. However, only 1% or less of T cells are actually infected, so other mechanisms than direct cytotoxicity have been invoked, including autoimmune destruction (see below).

Mac Macrophages and the related antigen-presenting cells, brain microglia, etc. are probably a main reservoir of HIV. They may also be the initial cell to become infected.

Transmission is still mainly by intercourse (heterosexual as well as homosexual) though in some areas infected blood from drug needles is more common. Not every exposure to HIV leads to infection, but as few as 10 virus particles are thought to be able to do so.

Pathology HIV is a lytic virus, but calculations suggest that uninfected as well as infected T cells die. A role has been proposed for autoimmunity against CD4, cytotoxicity by CD8 cells, cytokine imbalance, inappropriate apoptosis, cell fusion, soluble CD4 molecules, and many other scenarios.

Immunity The major antibody responses to HIV are against p24, p41, and gp120, but generally raised levels of Ig may occur, due to polyclonal B cell activation. A strong CD8 T response against HIV-infected cells persists throughout the asymptomatic phase of HIV infection, suggesting that these cells are the major effector mechanism keeping HIV replication in check. There is some evidence that these responses could be protective, based on vaccine trials in monkeys but the phenomenally high rate of antigenic variation makes all these responses less effective than they should be.

Therapy Early drugs used for treatment against HIV were inhibitors of viral reverse transcriptase, such as zidovudine (AZT). Treatment with a single drug provides only very short-term benefit as the virus mutates so fast that resistant strains soon emerge. However, the development of new families of drugs, for example against the HIV specific protease, allowed the introduction of multidrug therapy, in which patients are treated with three, four or even more different antivirals simultaneously. These regimes have seen some spectacular successes in the clinic, leading to disappearance of AIDS-associated infections, and undetectable levels of virus for over two years. However, it is too soon to say whether this approach ever results in permanent elimination of virus, and in any case the cost is prohibitive in most of the countries where HIV is common. Thus the requirement for an effective HIV vaccine remains acute, and several trials aimed especially at stimulating a strong cellular response are under way.

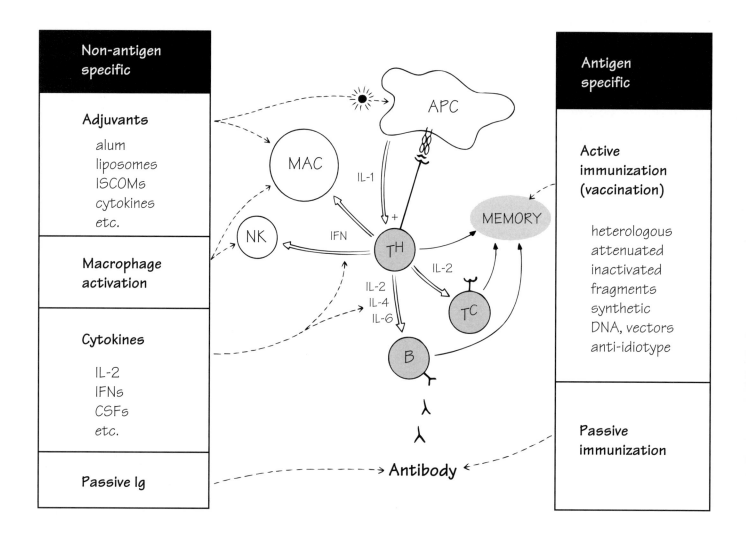

In most animals the combination of natural resistance and stimulation of adaptive responses by antigen is adequate to cope with common infections (otherwise the species would not survive!) However, the immune system does have its shortcomings, and some of these can be overcome by artificial means.

Natural immune mechanisms generally act, against a given challenge, either briskly or not at all. But there are times when they appear to be on the brink of success (e.g. against some tumours and parasites), and when it may be possible to tip the balance by **non-specific immunostimulation** (top left).

Adaptive immune responses, on the other hand, suffer from their initial slowness, so that high levels of antibody may arrive too late to prevent death or disability (e.g. tetanus, polio) even though surviving patients are resistant to reinfection. Here **specific immunization** is usually the answer; this may be **active** (top right), in which antigen is used to

safely generate immunological memory, aided in some cases by the boosting power of special non-specific stimulants or **adjuvants** (top left), or **passive**, in which preformed antibody is injected, with more rapid but short-lived effect. It is sometimes possible to increase immune responses by raising the level of the various soluble **mediators** (centre left).

Finally, when some component of the immune system is deficient (see Fig. 39), efforts can be made to correct this by **replacement** of hormones, enzymes, cytokines, cells, or organs. As knowledge grows, replacement of the defective **gene** will probably take the place of these temporizing measures. Meanwhile, new immunostimulants are constantly being reported, and the possibility that some apparently irrational remedy may benefit the immune system in ways at present unmeasurable, should never be hastily dismissed.

Adjuvants are materials which increase the response to an antigen given at the same time. One way in which many adjuvants work is by creating a slow-release depot of antigen, thus prolonging the time for which the immune system remains in contact with antigen. In addition, they contain substances which activate components of the innate immune system, and via this pathway also increase antigen presentation. Adjuvants include oil emulsions, metal salts (e.g. $Al(OH)_3$), and more recently synthetic lipid vesicles ('liposomes'), and lattices of saponin (ISCOMs). The most powerful adjuvants (e.g. Freund's Complete) are unfortunately too tissue-destructive for human use, and considerable efforts are being made to find safer adjuvants. Various defined fractions of mycobacterial cell walls (e.g. muramyl dipeptide) and plant substances (e.g. saponin) look promising, and several cytokines have also been shown to have adjuvant properties (IL-1, IL-2, IL-12, IFNγ).

Macrophage activation Mycobacteria (e.g. BCG), Corynebacteria, and other bacterial products (e.g. endotoxin) can increase many macrophage functions, including cytotoxicity against tumours. Many adjuvants also stimulate macrophages, and so do T cells (via cytokines), but the precise effects on macrophage function vary to some extent depending on the stimulus. Tumour necrosis factor (TNF) itself has so far been somewhat disappointing as an antitumour agent (see Fig. 31).

Replacement therapy In some cases of severe combined immunodeficiency, bone marrow grafting has restored function; where adenosine deaminase (ADA) is deficient, this enzyme may also be restored by blood transfusion. Thymus grafting has been effective in restoring T cell function in the Di George syndrome, and thymic hormones are being tried for a variety of T cell deficient states.

Cytokines Interferons, interleukins and other cytokines may have great potential for increasing the activity of their target cells. Natural killer cells are particularly susceptible to activation by both interferon and IL-2. INFα has proved useful in certain viral diseases and some rare tumours. Transfer factor, an extract of normal leucocytes, has apparently produced benefit in cases of infection due to T cell deficiency, but whether it acts specifically or non-specifically is still a controversial point.

Passive immunization

Antibody In patients already exposed to disease, passively transferred antiserum may be life-saving; examples are tetanus, hepatitis B, snakebite. Originally antisera were raised in horses, but the danger of serum sickness (see Fig. 34) makes convalescent human serum preferable. In patients with antibody deficiency, normal human gammaglobulin provides good protection against common infections. There should be a useful future for monoclonal antibodies against microbial antigens or toxins.

Active immunization ('vaccination')

The term 'vaccine' was introduced by Pasteur to commemorate Jenner's classic work with cowpox (vaccinia), but was extended by him to all agents used to induce specific immunity and mitigate the effects of subsequent infection. Vaccines are given as early as practical, taking into account the fact that the immune system is not fully developed in the first months of life, and that antibody passively acquired from the mother via the placenta and/or milk will specifically prevent the baby making his own response. In general this means a first injection at about 6 months, with subsequent boosts, but precise schedules may depend on the local prevalence of particular diseases, and can be found in specialized textbooks.

Living heterologous vaccines work by producing a milder but cross-protecting disease, the only common example being vaccinia, which has effectively allowed the elimination of smallpox.

Living attenuated viruses (measles, mumps, yellow fever, polio (Sabin), rubella) or bacteria (BCG) produce subclinical disease and usually excellent protection. Care is needed, however, in immunodeficient patients.

Inactivated vaccines are used where attenuation is not feasible; they include formalin-killed viruses such as rabies and influenza, and bacteria such as cholera and pertussis (whooping cough). Killed vaccines are safer but usually less effective than live ones, though some of them may have a useful adjuvant effect on other vaccines given with them (e.g. pertussis in the 'triple vaccine' with diphtheria and tetanus).

Toxoids are bacterial toxins (e.g. diphtheria, tetanus) inactivated with formalin but still antigenic.

Capsular polysaccharides induce some (primarily IgM) antibody against meningococcal, pneumococcal and haemophilus infection. However, the level and persistence of protective antibody can be greatly enhanced by coupling the polysaccharide to protein antigens, which stimulate a strong 'helper' response. Tetanus toxoid is frequently used for this purpose. These 'conjugate' vaccines are finding increasing use in the fight against bacterial meningitis.

Viral subunit vaccines. These are the first of the 'second generation' vaccines, in which the purified antigens are produced by recombinant DNA technology. So far only hepatitis A and B surface antigens have been produced in this way, but they provide a high (>90%) level of protection.

DNA, vectors An exciting new idea is to insert genes from one microbe into another less virulent one such as vaccinia or salmonella, which then behaves like a living vaccine for the desired antigen. If the vector has a large enough genome (e.g. BCG) multiple antigens could be introduced into a single vector, cutting down the need for repeated doses. Recently it has been found that DNA encoding for a protein antigen can simply be injected into the patient's muscle or skin and provoke an immune response — a totally unexpected result. One way to do this is to coat the DNA onto small gold particles, which are then fired under pressure into the skin — doing away with the need for needles. Vaccines making use of this 'particle-mediated' delivery system are currently being tried for a variety of infectious diseases and also for cancer.

42 Comparative sizes

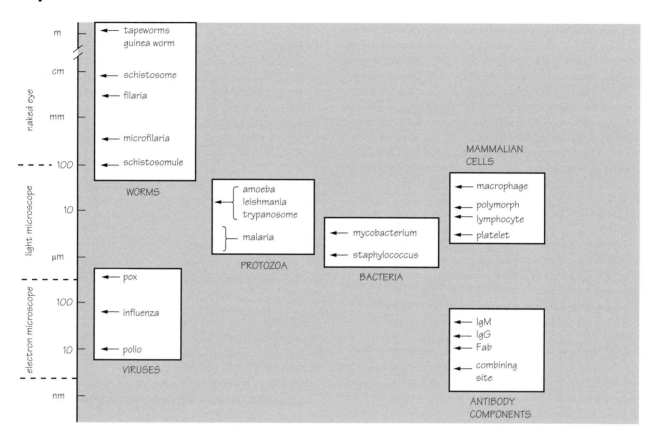

Comparative molecular weights

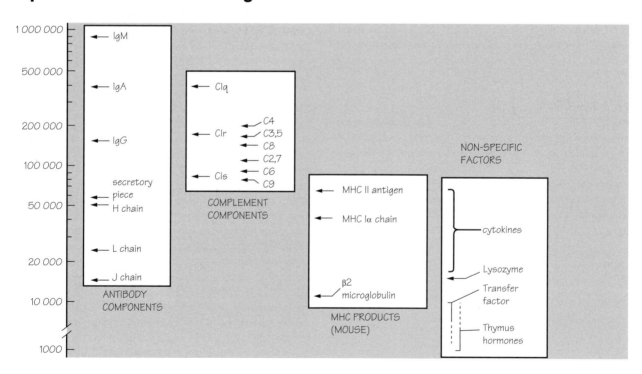

43 Landmarks in the history of immunology

1798	Jenner: vaccination against smallpox: the beginning of immunology
1881–5	Pasteur: attenuated vaccines (cholera, anthrax, rabies)
1882	Metchnikoff: phagocytosis (in starfish)
1888	Roux: Yersin: diphtheria antitoxin (antibody)
1890	Von Behring: passive protection (tetanus) by antibody
1891	Koch: delayed hypersensitivity (tuberculosis)
1893	Buchner: heat labile serum factor (complement)
1896	Widal: diagnosis by antibody (typhoid)
1897	Ehrlich: 'side chain' (receptor) theory
1900	Landsteiner: ABO groups in blood transfusion
1902	Portier & Richet: hypersensitivity
1903	Arthus: local anaphylaxis
1906	Von Pirquet: allergy
1910	Dale: histamine
1917–	Landsteiner: haptens, carriers and antibody specificity
1922	Fleming: lysozyme
1924	Glenny: adjuvants
1936	Gorer: transplantation antigens
1938	Tiselius & Kabat: antibodies as gammaglobulins
1943	Chase: transfer of delayed hypersensitivity by cells
1944–	Medawar: skin graft rejection as an immune response
1945	Coombs: antiglobulin test for red-cell autoantibody
1947	Owen: tolerance in cattle twins
1952	Bruton: agammaglobulinaemia
1953	Billingham, Brent & Medawar: neonatal induction of tolerance
1956	Glick: bursa dependence of antibody response
1956	Roitt & Doniach: autoantibodies in thyroid disease
1957	Isaacs & Lindenman: interferon
1958	Gell & Coombs: classification of hypersensitivities
1959	Porter; Edelman: enzyme cleavage of antibody molecule
1959	Gowans: lymphocyte recirculation
1959	Burnet: clonal selection theory
1960	Nowell: lymphocyte transformation (PHA)
1961–2	Miller; Good: thymus dependence of immune responses
1965	Di George: thymus deficiency
1966	David, Bloom & Bennett: macrophage activation by cytokines
1966–7	Claman; Davies; Mitchison: T–B cell co-operation
1968	Dausset: HLA
1969	McDevitt: Immune response genes
1971	Gershon: suppression by T cells
1974	Jerne: network theory of immune regulation
1975	Unanue; Antigen processing for Class II MHC
1975	Zinkernagel & Doherty; Bevan, Shevach: dual recognition by T Cells
1975	Köhler & Milstein: monoclonal antibodies from hybridomas
1976	Tonegawa: immunoglobulin gene rearrangement
1980	Smallpox eradicated
1981	AIDS recognized
1982	First recombinant subunit vaccine for Hepatitis B
1984–	Marrack, Davis, Hedrick: T cell receptor structure and genetics
1986–	Townsend, Braciale: Antigen processing for Class I MHC.
1986–	Coffman & Mosmann: T^{H1} and T^{H2} subsets
1987	Bjorkman: structure of MHC Class I molecule
1990	Wolff, Tang: DNA immunization
1993	Feldmann: anti-TNFα therapy for RA
1996	Wilson, Wiley: T cell receptor/MHC cocrystal

Some unsolved problems

AIDS: why do so many T cells die? Will a vaccine work?

Autoimmunity: is it all due to viruses?

Cancer: will immunology help?

Cytokines: (interleukins, interferons, growth factors): why so much overlap in function?

HLA and disease: how and why are they associated?

Human organ grafting: what are the critical antigens and will specific tolerance be possible?

Immunodeficiency: will gene therapy be the cure?

Macrophages: how do they recognize foreignness?

Networks: how important are they in regulating immune responses and can they be exploited to control them?

Psychoneuroimmunology: fact or fad?

T cells: how do suppressor T cells work? How can the same T cell receptor be selected negatively *and* positively?

Vaccination: will the parasite diseases succumb? How does the 'naked DNA' vaccine work?

Tolerance: how important is the thymus?

Hypermutation: what is the mechanism?

CD number	Function	Distribution
1a,b,c	Non-peptide antigen presentation	T, B, DC
2	Co-stimulation	T
3	Antigen-specific T cell activation	T
4	T cell co-stimulation	T, M, DC
5	Co-stimulation	T, some B
6	Adhesion/co-stimulation	T, some B
7	Co-stimulation/adhesion ??	T
8	Co-stimulation	T
9	Co-stimulation/ adhesion/activation	T, B, P, E
10	Endopeptidase	B, G, other ??
11a,b,c	Adhesion (integrin α chains)	T, B, M, DC, G
12	Not known	??
13	Aminopeptidase N	M, DC, G, E
14	LPS receptor	M
15	Adhesion (Lewis X)	M, G
16	Low affinity IgG receptor	M
17	Not known	Widespread
18	Adhesion (integrin β2 chain)	B, T, M, G
19	Co-stimulation	B
20	Co-stimulation	B
21	Complement receptor	B
22	Adhesion/co-stimulation	B
23	Low affinity IgE receptor	B
24	Adhesion ?	B, G
25	IL-2 receptor chain	T
26	Dipeptidyl peptidase	E
27	Co-stimulation	T, B
28	Co-stimulation	T
29	Adhesion (integrin β1)	Widespread
30	Co-stimulation	B
31	Adhesion	M, G, E
32	Low-affinity IgG receptor	M, G, P
33	Adhesion	M, G
34	Adhesion	E
35	Complement receptor	M, G
36	Scavenger receptor	M, P
37	Co-stimulation ??	T, B
38	ADP-ribosyl cyclase	T, B
39	Not known	B, ??
40	Co-stimulation	B, M, DC
41	Adhesion (integrin)	P
42a–d	Adhesion	T, P
43	Adhesion/anti-adhesion	T, B, M, DC, G
44	Adhesion/co-stimulation	T, B, M, DC, G
45, 45RA, 45RB, 45RC, 45RO	Co-stimulation, T cell memory marker	T, B
46	Complement regulator	Widespread
47	Adhesion	Widespread
48	Adhesion	Widespread
49a–f	Adhesion (integrin α1–6 chains)	Widespread
50	Adhesion (ICAM)	B, T, M, DC, G

CD number	Function	Distribution
51	Adhesion (integrin α chain)	P, E
52	Not known	T, B, M
53	Co-stimulation	T, B, M, G
54	Adhesion (ICAM)	Widespread
55	Complement regulation	Widespread
56	Adhesion	NK
57	Adhesion	NK, ??
58	Co-stimulation	B, M, DC, G, P, E
59	Complement regulation	Widespread
60a–c	Co-stimulation ???	P, E
61	Adhesion (integrin β3)	P, E
62E, 62L, 62P	Adhesion, homing	T, B, M, G, P, E
63	Not known	M, G, P, E
64	High-affinity IgG receptor	M
65	Adhesion ??	M, G
66a-f	Co-stimulation, adhesion	G
67	Alternative name for 66b	G
68	Lysosomal receptor	M
69	Co-stimulation, activation	T, M, G, P
70	Co-stimulation	B
71	Transferrin receptor	B, T
72	5 ligand	B
73	Ecto-5'-nucleotidase	B
74	Antigen processing (invariant chain)	T, B, M, DC
75	Cell adhesion	B
76	Not known	B
77	Apoptosis	B
78	Not assigned	
79a,b	Antigen specific activation	B
80	Co-stimulation	B, DC
81	Co-stimulation	T, B
82	Co-stimulation	T, B, M, G
83	Not known	B, DC
84	Not known	B, M
85	Not known	T, B, DC
86	Co-stimulation	B, M, DC
87	Urokinase plasminogen activator receptor	Widespread
88	Complement receptor	M, G
89	Fca receptor	M, G
90	Haemopoeisis (Thy 1)	T, B, E
91	α2-macroglobulin receptor	M
92	Not known	T, B, M, G
93	Not known	M, G, E
94	NK inhibitory receptor	NK
95	Apoptosis	T, B, E
96	Adhesion	T, NK
97	Adhesion	T, B, M, G
98	Amino acid transport, adhesion, cell activation	Widespread

CD number	Function	Distribution
99	Apoptosis	T, B, P.E
100	Co-stimulation	Widespread
101	Co-stimulation	M
102	Adhesion (ICAM)	??
103	Adhesion (integrin)	T, B
104	Adhesion (integrin)	T, B, E
105	TGF-co-receptor	E
106	Adhesion	E
107a,b	Not known (LAMP)	B, E
108	Not known	Widespread
109	Not known	T, E
110	Platelet production (TPO receptor)	P
111	Chemokine receptor	M
112	Chemokine receptor	M
113	Not assigned	
114	Haemopoeisis	G, P
115	M-CSF receptor	B, M
116	GM-CSF receptor	M, G
117	Haemopoesis	S
118	Not assigned	
119	IFNγ receptor	Widespread
120a,b	TNFα receptor	Widespread
121a,b	IL-1 receptor	Widespread
122	IL-2, IL-15 receptor	T, B
123	IL-3 receptor	Widespread
124	IL-4/IL-13 receptor	T, B
125	IL-5 receptor	B
126	IL-6 receptor	Widespread
127	IL-7 receptor	T
128	Chemokine receptor	M, G
130	IL-6, IL-11, and multiple other cytokine receptors	E
131	IL-3, IL-5, GM-CSF receptor	Widespread
132	IL-2, IL-4, IL-7, IL-9, L-15 receptor	T, B
133	Haemopoeisis (?)	Stem cells
134	Adhesion/co-stimulation	T
135	Haemopoeisis	Immature cells only
136	Differentiation	Immature cells only
137	Co-stimulation	T
138	Adhesion	T, B
139	Not known	Widespread
140	PDGF receptor	E
141	Blood clotting	E
142	Blood clotting	E
143	Angiotensin converting enzyme	E
144	Adhesion	E
145	Not known	E
146	Adhesion (?)	B, E
147	Adhesion (?)	Widespread
148	Activation (?)	Widespread
149	Reclassified as 47	
150	Co-stimulation	T, B
151	Adhesion	Widespread

CD number	Function	Distribution
152	Co-stimulation	T, B
153	Co-stimulation	T, B
154	Co-stimulation	T, B
155	Not known (poliovirus receptor)	T, E
156	Metalloproteinase	M, G
157	ADP-ribosyl cyclase	M, G
158a,b	NK inhibitory receptor	NK
159	NK inhibitory receptor	NK
160	Co-stimulation (?)	T, NK
161	NK inhibitory receptor	NK
162	Adhesion	Not known
163	Not known	Not known
164	Adhesion	Widespread
165	Adhesion	T, P
166	Adhesion	T, B, E

The distribution shows the major expression on the following cell types only:

T: T cells; B: B cells; M: monocyte/macrophage; G: granulocyte; P: platelets; E: endothelium; NK: natural killer cells; DC: dendritic cells; (?), ??: the distribution or function are still doubtful.

Further designations up to 247 have been assigned at the VIIth Workshop on Human Leukocyte Differentiation Antigens but full details are not yet available (see www. gryphon.jr2.ox.ac.uk)

Index

Numbers in **bold** type indicate the chapters in which principal references appear. Numbers indicate the chapter number not the page number.

ABO blood groups 37
Acute phase proteins 6
ADA deficiency 39
Adaptive immunity 1, 2
ADCC 9
Addison's disease 36
Adenoids 11
Adhesion molecules 6, 12, 14
Adjuvants 36, **41**
Adrenaline 33
Affinity **19**, 34
AFP 21, 31
Agammaglobulinaemia 39
Age, immunity and 39
Aggressins 27
AIDS 26, 39, **40**
Allelic exclusion 16
Allergy 33
Allograft 37
Allotype 16
Alternative pathway 5
Aluminium hydroxide 41
Amoeba 3, 29
Amphibians 3
Anaemia haemolytic 36
Anaphylaxis 33
Anaphylotoxin 5, 6
Ankylosing spondylitis 13
Antibody 2
    deficiency 39
    diversity 15
    response 18
    structure 16
    undesirable effects 32
Antigen **2**, 18
    division 31
    embryonic 31
    oral 21
    presentation 7, **17**, 18, 19
    sequestered 36
    suicide 21, 37, 38
    tumour specific 31
Antigenic variation 26, 29
Antihistamines 33
Anti-inflammatory drugs 33, 38
Antilymphocyte serum 38
Antiproliferative drugs 38
Apoptosis 9, 10
Arthritis, rheumatoid 34, 36
Arthropods 3
Arthus reaction 34
Ascorbic acid 8
Aspergillus 28
Asthma 33
Ataxia telengectasia 39
Atopy; atopic 33
Autoantibody 26, 27, 29, **36**
Autoimmune disease 1, **36**
Avidity 19
Azathioprine 38

B, factor 5
B cell *see* B lymphocyte
B lymphocyte 9, 18

activation, polyclonal 29, 36
    deficiency 39
Babesia 29
Bacteria 27
BALT 11
Basement membrane 34
Basophil 4, 20, **33**
BCG 31, 41
Beta (β)2 microglobulin 13
Birds 3
Blast cell, transformation 4, 9
Blood transfusion 37
Bone marrow 4, 10
    grafting 37, 41
Borrelia 27
Bruton O.C. 39
BSE 26
Burkitt's lymphoma 31
Burnet F.M. 21
Bursa of Fabricius 10

C, 1–9 (complement) 5
C-reactive protein 5, 6
Calcium 5, 33
Candidiasis 28
Capsule, bacterial 8, **27**
Carcino-embryonic antigen 31
Carrier 18
Catalase 8
Cathepsin 8
Cationic proteins 4, 8
Cell
    B 9
    K 9, 19, 25
    mast 2, 4, 6, **33**
    myeloid 4, 8
    NK 9, 31
    plasma 4, 9, 15
    stem 4
    T 9
Cell-mediated immunity 20
CGD 39
Chediak–Higashi disease 39
Chemokine 6, 23
Chemotaxis 6, 23
Chlorambucil 38
Chronic granulomatous disease 39
CJD 26
Class, immunoglobulin 16
Classical pathway 5
Clonal
    elimination 21, 38
    proliferation 18
    selection 18, 20
Clone, hybrid 4
Clonorchis 30
Clotting, blood 6
Coley 31
Combining site 16, 19
Complement 2, 5, 6, 34
    deficiencies 39
    receptors 5
Complex, immune **19**, 34
CON A 9
Concomitant immunity 30, 31
Constant region (Ig) 15, 16
Contact sensitivity 35

Coombs R.R.A. 32
Cooperation 2, 18
Copper 39
Corals 3
Corneal graft 37
Corynebacteria 41
Co-stimulation 14
Crohn's disease 35
Cross-reaction 36
Cryoprecipitation 19
Cryptosporidium 29
CSF 4, 23
Cyclic AMP, GMP 33
Cyclophosphamide 38
Cyclosporin A 38
Cyclostomes 3
Cytokines 23
Cytostasis 31
Cytotoxicity 20
    antibody-dependent 19

D, factor 5
DAF 5
Delayed hypersensitivity **20**, 31, 35
Dendritic cell 4, **7**
Determinant, antigenic 19
Dextran, dextran sulphate 9
Di George syndrome 39
Diabetes 36
Diffuse intravascular coagulation 34
Diphtheria 27
Domain, Ig 12, 16
Drugs, and autoimmunity 36
    and immunosuppression 38, 39
Dysgenesis, reticular 39

Echinoderms 3
Emotions 24, 33
Endoplasmic reticulum 8, 15
Endothelial cell 7
Endotoxic shock 32
Endotoxin 27, 34
Enhancement 21, 31, 38
Eosinophil 4, 8, 30, 35
Epithelioid cell 20, 35
Epstein–Barr virus (EBV) 26
Exotoxin 27

Fab fragment of Ig 16
Factor B, D 5
Farmer's lung 28
Fasciola 30
Fc fragment of Ig 16
Feedback, antibody 18
Fibrosis 6, 35
Filaria 30
Fishes 3
Flagella 27
Fetal immunization 21
    liver 10
Fetus, as graft 37
Food 21
Freund's adjuvant 41
Fungi 28

Gell P.G.H. 32
Gene,
    immunoglobulin 12, 13, **15**

Gene (contd)
    MHC receptor   12, 13
    T cell receptor   12, 14
Germ line   14, **15**
Germinal centre   11, 18
Giant cell   20, 35
Golgi apparatus   8, 17
Goodpasture's syndrome   34
Grafting   37
Granulocyte   4
Granuloma   6, 20, **35**
Gut, lymphoid tissue   11
GVH (graft-versus-host)   37

Haemolytic anaemia   36
Haemopoiesis   4
Hagfish   3
Hapten   18
Hassal's corpuscle   10
Help   2, 18
Helper (T) cell   9, 18
Hepatitis virus   26, 34
Herpes virus   26
Histamine   6, 33
Histoplasmosis   28
HLA, H2   13
Hybrid clone   4
Hydrogen peroxide   8
Hydrophobic forces   8, 19
Hypersensitivity   1, **32**

I region   13
Idiotypes   22
Ig see Immunoglobulin
Immune adherence   7
Immune complex   **19**, 34
Immune response   1, 18, 20
Immunization
    active   1, 41
    passive   41
Immunity   2
    cell mediated   20
    concomitant   30, 31
Immunodeficiency   39
Immunoglobulin (Ig)
    classes, etc.   16
    deficiency   39
    function   16, 19
    superfamily   12
    IgA   16, 26, 27
    IgD   16
    IgE   16, 30, 33
    IgG   16, 19
    IgM   16
Immunostimulation   31, **41**
Immunosuppression   26, 29, 38
Infection, immunity to   25–30
    opportunistic   29
Inflammation, acute   **6**, 33, 34
    chronic   35
Influenza   26
Insect bites   33
Interferon   2, 23, **26**, 31
Interleukins   20, 23
Invariant chain   17
Iron   8, 39

J chain   16
J region   15
Jones–Mote hypersensitivity   35

K cell   9, 19, 25
KAF   5
Kappa chain   16
Kidney grafting   37

Killer T cell   20
Kupffer cell   7, 34
Kuru   26

Lactoferrin   8
LAF   20, 23
Lambda chain   16
Lamprey   3
Langerhans cell   7
Lectins   9
Leishmaniasis   29
Leprosy   27
Leukotrienes   6, 34
Light chain   16
Linkage disequilibrium   13
Lipopolysaccharide   9, 27
Liposome   41
Liver, fetal   10
LPS   9, 27
Lung   11
Ly antigens   9
Lymph node   11
Lymphocyte   2, **9**
    see also B lymphocyte, T lymphocyte
Lymphokines   20, 23
Lymphotoxin   20, 23, 31
Lysis   5, 19, 25
Lysosome   8, 9, 13
Lysozyme   2, 8, **27**
LyT antigens   9

M cell   11
M Protein   27
Macrophage   2, 7, 8, 18, 20, 21, 35
    activation   31, 41
Magnesium   5
Malaria   29
Malnutrition   39
MALT   11
Mantoux test   35
Marginal zone   11
Mast cell   2, 4, 6, **33**
MBP   5, 39
Measles   26, 39, 41
Memory   2, 18, 20
Mesangium   7, 34
Metchnikoff E.   3
MHC   **13**, 37
Microfilament   8
Microglia   7
Micro-organisms, immunity to   25
Microtubule   8
MIF   20
Mixed lymphocyte reaction   37
Molluscs   3
Monoclonal antibody   9, 16
Monocyte   4, 6, 7, 35
Multiple sclerosis   26
Muramidase   2, 8, **27**
Mutation, somatic   **15**, 36
Myasthenia gravis   36
Mycobacteria   27
Mycoplasma   26
Myeloid cell   4, 8
Myeloma   16
Myeloperoxidase   8

Narcolepsy   13
Natural immunity   1, 2
Networks   18, 21, 22
Nezelof syndrome   39
Niridazole   38
Nitric oxide   8
NK cell   2, **9**, 31

Non-self   1, 21, 36
Nurse cells   10

Onchocerciasis   30
Oncogenes   26, 31
Opportunistic infection   29
Opsonization   **8**, 25
Osteoclast   7

Papain   16
Paracortex   11
PCA test   33
PEG   19
Pepsin   16
Peptidoglycan   27
Perforin   20
Permeability, vascular   **6**, 33
Pernicious anaemia   36
Peyer's patch   11
PHA   9
Phagocytosis   7, **8**
Phagosome   8
Pinocytosis   8
Plasma cell   4, 9, 15, 18
Plasma exchange   38
Platelet   4, 6, 7, 32, 33
Pneumococcus   27
Pneumocystis   28, 29
PNP   9, 39
Pokeweed mitogen   9
Polio virus   26
Pollen   33
Polyarteritis nodosa   34
Poly-Ig receptor   12
Polymorph   4, 6, 7, 8, 32, 34
Polysaccharides   27, 41
Post-capillary venule   10
Pox virus   26
PPD   9
Pregnancy   37
Premunition   29
Presentation (antigen)   2, 7, 17, 18, 20
Prion   26
Privileged sites (graft)   37
Programmed cell death   9, 10
Properdin   5
Prostaglandins   6
Protozoa   3, 29

Qa antigens   13

Rabies vaccine   41
Reactive lysis   19
Reagin, reaginic antibody   33
Receptor
    Fc   8, 9, 33
    C3   8, 9
Relapsing fever   27
Replacement therapy   41
Reptiles   3
Restriction endonucleases   3
Retiarian therapy   38
Reticular cell   7
Reticular dysgenesis   39
Reticulo-endothelial system   7
Retroviruses   26, 31, 40
Rhesus blood groups   37
Rheumatoid arthritis   34, 36
Rickettsia   26
Ringworm   28
RNA, double-stranded   41
Rosette forming cell   9

Salmonella   27
Sarcoidosis   35

Index   95

Schistosomiasis 30
Schwartzmann reaction 34
SCID 39
Secondary response 18, 20
Secretory piece 16
Self 1, 21, 36
Serotonin 33
Serum sickness 34
Severe combined immunodeficiency 39
Sequestered antigens 36
Sequestration 25, 35
Sharks 3
Shigella 27
Skin 11, 25, 30
SLE 34, 36
Smallpox 26, 41
Somatic mutation **15**, 36
Snakebite 41
Spleen 11
Sponges 3
Staphylococcus 27
Stem cell 4
Steroids 28, 38
Streptococcus 27, 35
Subclass (Ig) 16
Suicide, antigen 21, 37, 38
Superantigen 14, 21
Superoxide 8
Suppressor T cell 9, 18, 21
Syngraft 37
Syphilis 27, 36

T3, T4, T8, T$_i$ 14
T cell *see* T lymphocyte
T lymphocyte 9
  cytotoxic 9, 20
  helper 9, 18
  receptor **14**, 18, 20
  suppressor 9, 18, 21
  surveillance 31
TAP 17
Tapeworms 30
TCGF 20, 23
Temporal arteritis 34
Tetanus 27, 41
TGFβ 23
Theileria 29
Thrombocytopenia 36
Thy 1 (theta) 9, 12
Thymosin 4, **10**, 39
Thymus 10
  deficiency 39
  grafting 41
Thyroiditis 32, 34, 36
Tissue typing 37
TL antigen 9
Tolerance **21**, 38
Toll receptor 3
Tonsil 11
Toxin 27
Toxoid 41
Toxoplasmosis 29
Trachoma 26
Traffic, cell 6

Transfer factor 28, 31, 41
Trypanosome 29
Tuberculin response 20
Tuberculosis 27
Tumour necrosis factor 23, 31
Tumours **31**, 39, 41
Tunicates 3
Typhoid 27
Typhus 26
Typing, tissue 37

UV light 11, 31

Vaccination 1, 22, **41**
Van der Waals forces 19
Variable region (Ig) 15, 16
Vascular permeability **6**, 33, 34, 35
Vasoamines 6, 33
Veiled cell 7
Viruses, immunity to 26

Wiskott–Aldrich syndrome 39
Worms 3, 30

X-linked genes 39
X-rays 4, 37, 38
Xenograft 37

Yellow fever 26
Yolk sac 10

Zinc 39
Zoonoses 26, 27